David Woodland
1201 Hague Ave
St Paul, MN 55104

D10111414

Steven I. Pfeiffer, PhD, ABPP
*Editor*

# Outcome Assessment in Residential Treatment

*More pre-publication*
*REVIEWS, COMMENTARIES, EVALUATIONS . . .*

"*Outcome Assessment in Residential Treatment*, edited by Steven I. Pfeiffer, is a major surprise in a research area too long bereft of adequate scholarship. Taken collectively, the selected papers describe how research in residential treatment can be both academic *and* practical. An erudite review of the extant literature sets the stage for Rex Green and Frederick Newman's brilliant exposition of their five steps and eleven criteria for conducting field based research. Their elaboration of Step I: Decide What to Measure, and Step II: Identify Unwanted Effects, will describe how the the reader can conduct research that is both clinically useful and academically rigorous.

Patrick Zimmerman presents a brief, useful and critical description of a wide variety of outcome measures currently in use. . . . Paul LeBuffe and Steven Pfeiffer provide information that can aid researchers to appropriately use, and accurately interpret, data generated by the Devereux Scales of Mental Disorder. Frequently, logistics and institutional climate are the greatest barriers to quality field based research. All of the teachings of the other authors would be wasted by a researcher who does not understand Pfeiffer and Shott's treatise on working within an institutional setting."

**Robert B. Bloom, PhD**
*Executive Director*
*Jewish Children's Bureau of Chicago*

The Haworth Press, Inc.

# Outcome Assessment
# in Residential Treatment

# Outcome Assessment in Residential Treatment

Steven I. Pfeiffer, PhD, ABPP
Editor

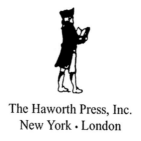

The Haworth Press, Inc.
New York · London

*Outcome Assessment in Residential Treatment* has also been published as *Residential Treatment for Children & Youth*, Volume 13, Number 4 1996.

The development, preparation, and publication of this work has been undertaken with great care. However, the publisher, employees, editors, and agents of The Haworth Press and all imprints of The Haworth Press, Inc., including The Haworth Medical Press and Pharmaceutical Products Press, are not responsible for any errors contained herein or for consequences that may ensue from use of materials or information contained in this work. Opinions expressed by the author(s) are not necessarily those of The Haworth Press, Inc.

The Haworth Press, Inc., 10 Alice Street, Binghamton, NY 13904-1580 USA

**Library of Congress Cataloging-in-Publication Data**

Outcome assessment in residential treatment / Steven I. Pfeiffer.
      p. cm.
   Includes bibliographical references and index.
   ISBN 1-56024-839-4 (alk. paper)
      1. Child psychotherapy–Residential treatment. 2. Outcome assessment (Medical care)
I. Pfeiffer, Steven I.
RJ504.5.O98 1996
618.92'8914–dc20                                                            96-20075
                                                                                CIP

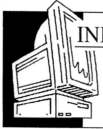

# INDEXING & ABSTRACTING

Contributions to this publication are selectively indexed or abstracted in print, electronic, online, or CD-ROM version(s) of the reference tools and information services listed below. This list is current as of the copyright date of this publication. See the end of this section for additional notes.

- *Applied Social Sciences Index & Abstracts (ASSIA) (Online: ASSI via Data-Star) (CD-Rom: ASSIA Plus),* Bowker-Saur Limited, Maypole House, Maypole Road, East Grinstead, West Sussex RH19 1HH, England

- *Cambridge Scientific Abstracts,* Health & Safety Science *Abstracts,* Environmental Routenet (accessed via INTERNET), 7200 Wisconsin Avenue #601, Bethesda, MD 20814

- *Child Development Abstracts & Bibliography,* University of Kansas, 2 Bailey Hall, Lawrence, KS 66045

- *CNPIEC Reference Guide: Chinese National Directory of Foreign Periodicals,* P.O. Box 88, Beijing, People's Republic of China

- *Criminal Justice Abstracts,* Willow Tree Press, 15 Washington Street, 4th Floor, Newark, NJ 07102

- *Criminology, Penology and Police Science Abstracts,* Kugler Publications, P.O. Box 11188, 1001 GD Amsterdam, The Netherlands

- *Exceptional Child Education Resources (ECER), (online through DIALOG and hard copy),* The Council for Exceptional Children, 1920 Association Drive, Reston, VA 22091

- *Family Studies Database (online and CD/ROM),* Peters Technology Transfer, 306 East Baltimore Pk., 2nd Floor, Media, PA 19063

- *IBZ International Bibliography of Periodical Literature,* Zeller Verlag GmbH & Co., P.O.B. 1949, d-49009, Osnabruck, Germany

- *Index to Periodical Articles Related to Law,* University of Texas, 727 East 26th Street, Austin, TX 78705

(continued)

- *International Bulletin of Bibliography on Education*, Proyecto B.I.B.E./Apartado 52, San Lorenzo del Escorial, Madrid, Spain

- *INTERNET ACCESS (& additional networks) Bulletin Board for Libraries ("BUBL"), coverage of information resources on INTERNET, JANET, and other networks.*
  - JANET X.29: UK.AC.BATH.BUBL or 00006012101300
  - TELNET: BUBL.BATH.AC.UK or 138.38.32.45 login 'bubl'
  - Gopher: BUBL.BATH.AC.UK (138.32.32.45). Port 7070
  - World Wide Web: http: / / www.bubl.bath.ac.uk./BUBL/ home.html
  - NISSWAIS: telnetniss.ac.uk (for the NISS gateway)
  The Andersonian Library, Curran Building, 101 St. James Road, Glasgow G4 ONS, Scotland

- *Mental Health Abstracts (online through DIALOG)*, IFI/Plenum Data Company, 3202 Kirkwood Highway, Wilmington, DE 19808

- *National Clearinghouse on Child Abuse & Neglect*, 10530 Rosehaven Street, Suite 400, Fairfax, VA 22030-2840

- *Psychological Abstracts (PsycINFO)*, American Psychological Association, P.O. Box 91600, Washington, DC 20090-1600

- *Sage Family Studies Abstracts (SFSA)*, Sage Publications, Inc., 2455 Teller Road, Newbury Park, CA 91320

- *Social Planning/Policy & Development Abstracts (SOPODA)*, Sociological Abstracts, Inc., P.O. Box 22206, San Diego, CA 92192-0206

- *Social Work Abstracts*, National Association of Social Workers, 750 First Street NW, 8th Floor, Washington, DC 20002

- *Sociological Abstracts (SA)*, Sociological Abstracts, Inc., P.O. Box 22206, San Diego, CA 92192-0206

- *Sociology of Education Abstracts*, Carfax Publishing Company, P.O. Box 25, Abingdon, Oxfordshire OX14 3UE, United Kingdom

- *Special Educational Needs Abstracts*, Carfax Information Systems, P.O. Box 25, Abingdon, Oxfordshire OX14 3UE, United Kingdom

- *Violence and Abuse Abstracts: A Review of Current Literature on Interpersonal Violence (VAA)*, Sage Publications, Inc., 2455 Teller Road, Newbury Park, CA 91320

(continued)

# SPECIAL BIBLIOGRAPHIC NOTES

*related to special journal issues (separates)*
*and indexing/abstracting*

☐ indexing/abstracting services in this list will also cover material in any "separate" that is co-published simultaneously with Haworth's special thematic journal issue or DocuSerial. Indexing/abstracting usually covers material at the article/chapter level.

☐ monographic co-editions are intended for either non-subscribers or libraries which intend to purchase a second copy for their circulating collections.

☐ monographic co-editions are reported to all jobbers/wholesalers/approval plans. The source journal is listed as the "series" to assist the prevention of duplicate purchasing in the same manner utilized for books-in-series.

☐ to facilitate user/access services all indexing/abstracting services are encouraged to utilize the co-indexing entry note indicated at the bottom of the first page of each article/chapter/contribution.

☐ this is intended to assist a library user of any reference tool (whether print, electronic, online, or CD-ROM) to locate the monographic version if the library has purchased this version but not a subscription to the source journal.

☐ individual articles/chapters in any Haworth publication are also available through the Haworth Document Delivery Services (HDDS).

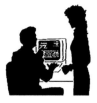

# Outcome Assessment in Residential Treatment

## CONTENTS

## ABOUT THE EDITOR

**Steven I. Pfeiffer, PhD, ABPP,** is Professor of Psychology in Psychiatry at the University of Pennsylvania Medical School and is currently Director of Behavioral Health for Genesis Health Ventures in Kennett Square, PA. For eight years he was Executive Director of the Devereux Foundation Institute of Clinical Training & Research in Devon, PA. The author of *Assessing Mental Health Treatment Outcomes* and *Clinical Child Psychology: An Introduction to Theory, Research and Practice*, Dr. Pfeiffer has also written several monographs and book chapters and more than 80 journal articles. He has been Editor of *Child & Adolescent Mental Health Care*, Guest Editor for *School Psychology Review*, and has served on the editorial boards of numerous other journals. He is a member of the American Academy of School Psychology, the American Association of Children's Residential Centers, and the American Psychological Association.

# Foreword

It is not news that American society has moved to a conservative position with a vengeance, and that Residential Treatment Centers need to reposition themselves accordingly. The national mandate is toward cost effectiveness, no longer personal growth, and we are expected to show results that justify our high cost.

Studies are complex, with subtle components such as the expense to society of the problems at home and on the streets. However, the RTCs are not required to solve the problem of our children going back to unchanged families and unchanged streets. Our contribution is limited to outcome studies of our residential work, which is complex enough.

We start at a disadvantage: the conservative stereotype that such youth cannot be helped at any cost. In fact they are hard to help, as is measuring the gains. Character change is at best slow. RTCs can almost always stop misbehavior readily enough; most of our children and youth can survive going home for short vacations after only a month or two. But the basic elements of residential treatment; education, psychotherapy, and parenting all change slowly. Growing maturity of thought and emotions are intangible, difficult to measure, and easy to overlook in light of an occasional glaring failure. However, the greatest challenge is the increasing psychological and social damage in our residential population. We are increasingly working with psychotic children and street kids, products of the culture of violence, the drug scene, and of gangs, who are especially mistrustful because of the anomie of the culture of poverty.

RTCs have an advantage that outweighs all these problems: we know we can usually help, given time and funding. Valid and reliable documenting is the only real problem. Proper outcome studies directly benefit the RTC staff to see beyond the daily drudgery and catastrophes to long term goals. This encouragement then carries into the Individual Education Plan meetings; they can present their long term gains and hopes for the future,

[Haworth co-indexing entry note]: "Foreword." Northrup, Gordon. Co-published simultaneously in *Residential Treatment for Children & Youth* (The Haworth Press, Inc.) Vol. 13, No. 4, 1996, pp. xv-xvi; and: *Outcome Assessment in Residential Treatment* (ed: Steven I. Pfeiffer) The Haworth Press, Inc., 1996, pp. xi-xii. Single or multiple copies of this article are available from The Haworth Document Delivery Service [1-800-342-9678, 9:00 a.m. - 5:00 p.m. (EST). E-mail address: getinfo@haworth.com].

(and so speak indirectly to the question of cost effectiveness) rather than just offering anecdotes of good behavior.

Outcome studies may seem a long way from our day-to-day therapeutic work, not our expertise, daunting, and difficult. True, careful work and statistical documentation are needed, but not large studies, and it is in fact best to start small. What is needed is the right guide. In this group of articles you will find practical, detailed and experienced advice on how to carry out studies that will benefit both the RTCs and the field. I hope you decide to proceed.

*Gordon Northrup, MD*
*Editor*

# Preface

Because residential treatment centers (RTCs), psychiatric hospitals and other behavioral healthcare settings are increasingly being asked to document their effectiveness, it is essential for providers of mental health care services to demonstrate the efficacy and cost-effectiveness of the services they provide. Displaced by demands for public accountability, public trust is no longer guaranteed. Various stakeholders–including professional peer groups, regulatory agencies, and market forces–are demanding verification of treatment effectiveness.

This pressure to document treatment outcomes makes self-evaluation essential to the continued existence of RTCs and psychiatric hospitals. Treatment outcome assessment provides an opportunity to understand the relative effects of specific interventions or procedures on the quality and effectiveness of mental health care. Treatment outcome assessment seeks to elucidate which therapeutic components contribute to the goals and objectives of the program and which may require modification, radical revision, or even elimination.

Today's healthcare providers must demonstrate that their planned treatment is necessary and active rather than simply custodial. Accurate information about the outcomes of care is essential for demonstrating that specific services are beneficial, cost-effective and well-received by the client. Outcome studies evaluate the impact a treatment program has on a client's clinical status, psychosocial and educational functioning, and provide an objective yardstick for the payers' evaluation of the quality of care provided. They also provide RTCs and psychiatric treatment facilities with an opportunity to document treatment successes and better understand which factors (within the child or adolescent, family, environment, treatment setting, and combinations therein) predict successful outcome. With such objective data, we are in a position to influence government and indus-

[Haworth co-indexing entry note]: "Preface." Pfeiffer, Steven I. Co-published simultaneously in *Residential Treatment for Children & Youth* (The Haworth Press, Inc.) Vol. 13, No. 4, 1996, pp. xvii-xviii; and: *Outcome Assessment in Residential Treatment* (ed: Steven I. Pfeiffer) The Haworth Press, Inc., 1996, pp. xiii-xiv. Single or multiple copies of this article are available from The Haworth Document Delivery Service [1-800-342-9678, 9:00 a.m. - 5:00 p.m. (EST). E-mail address: getinfo@haworth.com].

*xiii*

try, enhance public awareness of the needs of severely disturbed children and youth, and validate the usefulness of intensive psychiatric treatment.

The articles that make up this volume all argue that carefully designed treatment outcome research provides clear, program-specific data about the effectiveness and utility of our planned interventions. Without such data, the RTC or hospital administrator cannot hope to monitor or judge the effectiveness or value of clinical activities and therefore cannot adjust or improve therapeutic programs. Our hope is that the articles in this volume provide you with an appreciation of the value of treatment outcome assessment, specific strategies and techniques to initiate an outcomes project, and guidelines to ensure that your undertaking is a success.

*Steven I. Pfeiffer, PhD, ABPP*
*Director of Behavioral Health*
*Genesis Health Ventures*
*Kennett Square, PA*

# Introduction to Treatment Outcome: Historical Perspectives and Current Issues

Sarah I. Pratt, PhD
Kevin L. Moreland, PhD

**SUMMARY.** Outcome research on child and adolescent mental health services serves many important purposes, the most important of which is to improve upon the efficacy of techniques that may be used to alleviate the suffering of countless troubled youngsters. The current body of research in this area is small compared to the body of research on the outcomes of adult psychotherapy, perhaps because, historically, the treatment of childhood mental disorders has not received as much attention. Meta-analyses of outcome studies conducted over the past twenty years have concluded that research has demonstrated the efficacy of child and adolescent psychotherapy; however, recent evaluations of these meta-analyses have warned that most studies have included features that may not be generalizable to treatment as actually practiced in clinical settings. Measuring and defining improvement in any population is complicated and there is, as yet, no consensus on standards. For several reasons, conducting research on children and adolescents can be particularly problematic. Although significant strides have been made in child and adolescent mental health care, further research must include standardization of measures of improvement and finer-grained analyses of a greater number of the variables that may influence the efficacy of treatment. *[Article copies available from The Haworth Document Delivery Service: 1-800-342-9678. E-mail address: getinfo@haworth.com]*

---

Sarah I. Pratt and Kevin L. Moreland are affiliated with the Department of Psychology at Fordham University.

The authors may be written at the Department of Psychology, Fordham University, 441 East Fordham Road, Bronx, NY 10458-5198.

[Haworth co-indexing entry note]: "Introduction to Treatment Outcome: Historical Perspectives and Current Issues." Pratt, Sarah I., and Kevin L. Moreland. Co-published simultaneously in *Residential Treatment for Children & Youth* (The Haworth Press, Inc.) Vol. 13, No. 4, 1996, pp. 1-27; and: *Outcome Assessment in Residential Treatment* (ed: Steven I. Pfeiffer) The Haworth Press, Inc., 1996, pp. 1-27. Single or multiple copies of this article are available from The Haworth Document Delivery Service [1-800-342-9678, 9:00 a.m. - 5:00 p.m. (EST). E-mail address: getinfo@haworth.com].

Progress in the diagnosis, understanding and treatment of child and adolescent psychopathology has advanced considerably in recent years. Many researchers complain that outcome research on child and adolescent mental health services, particularly hospital treatment, lags behind research on adult treatment (Casey & Berman, 1985; Colson, Cornsweet, Murphy, O'Malley, Hyland, McPharland, & Coyne, 1991; Cornsweet, 1990; Klinge, Piggott, Knitter, & O'Donnell, 1986; Gabel & Shindledecker, 1990). Throughout history, progress in the treatment of adult psychopathology has outpaced that of children and adolescents (Cornsweet, 1990; Zimmerman, 1990). Until the late 1800s, disturbed children were often labeled delinquent, and frustrated parents customarily sent them to foster homes and other custodial institutions. Such facilities emphasized work and conformity and the children placed there generally were not expected to become productive, well-functioning members of society.

During the early 1900s, many new hospitals designed for the specialized care of adult psychiatric disorders opened. Twenty years later, the first children's psychiatric units were established at Bellevue, the Franklin School, Allentown State Hospital, and Kings Park State Hospital. The first all-adolescent units appeared in the late 1930s; however, until the 1950s, convention held that troubled adolescents were generally too aggressive and destructive for inpatient psychiatric care and therefore should be placed in facilities that emphasized strong discipline (Zimmerman, 1990). Services designed specifically for children and adolescents were not widely available until the 1950s, and the practice of treating disturbed children and adolescents in specialized units of hospitals became widespread only in the 1960s (Cornsweet, 1990). Therefore, it should perhaps come as little surprise that evaluations of the effectiveness of therapies designed specifically to treat child psychopathology would be lacking compared with assessments of adult treatment.

Heightened awareness of the impact of mental illness on society and the economy has increased concern about the effectiveness and cost of mental health services (Kazdin, 1990). Mental health care coverage, although increasingly scarce, represents a significant cost to businesses. In the late 1980s, the cost of mental health care was rising at a rate of 27% a year, making it the fastest rising health care cost (Moreland, Fowler, & Honaker, 1994). The US House of Representatives' Office of Technology Assessment reported in 1986 that 7.5 million children in the United States were experiencing an emotional, behavioral or developmental problem, and estimated that only 20-30% were receiving treatment, while even fewer were receiving treatment that was deemed adequate (cited in Rog, 1992).

Fiscal constraints have often caused policymakers to focus on reducing mental health care costs by reducing services, while minimizing the importance of evaluating outcomes achieved by therapeutic interventions (Davis & Frank, 1992). This is probably penny-wise and pound-foolish (cf. Yokley, Coleman, & Yates, 1990). Failing to provide care may have lasting adverse consequences, not only for the children receiving treatment but also for their families and society at large. Many dysfunctions that present in childhood and adolescence can either continue into adulthood essentially unchanged or metamorphose into adult psychopathology (Kazdin, 1993b; Cornsweet, 1990). If childhood disorders are not addressed, their severity may increase, resulting in greater cost in the long run (Berman & Austad, 1991). Untreated cases of childhood conduct disorder, for example, may cost society a great deal owing to delinquent acts committed in adulthood (Day, Pal, & Goldberg, 1994).

Outcome research will demonstrate to third party payers that treatment for troubled children and adolescents is more cost-effective, in the long run, than no treatment (Vermillion & Pfeiffer, 1993). However, the purpose of conducting outcome research extends beyond evaluating the general question of whether psychotherapy is effective. An obvious goal of outcome research should be to improve the quality and efficacy of treatment in order to reduce suffering in children and adolescents. Detailed studies of outcome will delineate which treatments are most effective for which disorders, and which factors tend to reliably predict favorable versus unfavorable outcome (Kazdin, 1990; Vermillion & Pfeiffer, 1993). Therefore, increased knowledge about outcomes may ultimately influence initial choice of treatment (Kazdin, 1993b). Outcome research serves as an important source of information for the design of prevention programs for at-risk children and adolescents (Kazdin, 1993b). Positive results obtained from outcome studies should also increase public awareness of the value of psychiatric treatment and thereby influence public policy regarding mental health care services.

## FINDINGS OF OUTCOME RESEARCH ON CHILD AND ADOLESCENT PSYCHOTHERAPY CONDUCTED TO DATE

An early review of child psychotherapy by Levitt (1957) called into question the efficacy of psychotherapy in much the same way that Eysenck's controversial review of adult psychotherapy had in 1952. In his evaluation of studies of child psychotherapy outcomes, Levitt (1957) found no evidence to support the assertion that treated children fared substantially better than untreated children. Several criticisms have been leveled against Levitt's methodology and conclusions. For example, the studies he reviewed included individuals whose ages ranged widely: from preschool through twenty-one years of age (Kazdin, 1990). Also, his untreated group consisted solely of children who were followed up after dropping out of treatment (Weisz, Weiss, & Bononberg, 1992). Levitt apparently failed to consider that the dropouts may have been qualitatively different from the children who remained in treatment, therefore making them inappropriate as controls. Finally, in Levitt's review, improvement was assessed by therapist ratings alone, without assessments by parents, or the patients themselves (Kazdin, 1990). It is now well known that assessments of improvement can vary widely depending on the source of the evaluation (Achenbach, 1994; Lachar & Kline, 1994; Casey & Berman, 1985).

Most recent meta-analyses[1] have found that treating children and adolescents yields improvement that is unlikely to occur simply as a function of time (Kazdin, 1993a; Casey & Berman, 1985; Weisz, Weiss, Alicke, & Klotz, 1987; Blotcky, Dimperio, & Gossett, 1984; Pfeiffer & Strzelecki, 1990). Recent meta-analyses collectively evaluating hundreds of outcome studies of child and adolescent mental health services have found significant positive effects of psychotherapy for children and adolescents, estimating that children who receive treatment function better than between 76%-81% of non-treated children (Casey & Berman, 1985; Weisz et al., 1987; Weisz et al., 1992). These findings are similar to the results obtained in recent meta-analyses of outcome studies of adult psychotherapy (Crits-Christoph, 1992; Shadish, Montgomery, Wilson, Wilson, Bright, & Okwumabua, 1993).

### Speculations About Outcomes from Predictor Variables

Several of these meta-analyses have attempted to identify predictor variables which may inform clinicians regarding choice of technique, nature and composition of treatment, expected course of therapy and/or hospitalization, and level of expectation for favorable outcome. These have included age, intelligence, gender, severity of dysfunction, and family functioning. Meta-analysts have reached substantial agreement on the effects of some of these variables, but remain divided on the impact of others.

Researchers appear to have reached a fair degree of consensus regarding the negative implications of organic brain dysfunction and severe "functional" diagnoses, antisocial behavior, and bizarre symptomatology. Not surprisingly, children who present a healthier clinical picture tend to have more favorable outcomes (Kolko, 1992; Blotcky et al., 1984; Pfeiffer & Strzelecki, 1990; Gossett, 1985).

There is also general agreement that healthy family functioning and supportive after-care services lead to significantly better outcomes (Blotcky et al., 1984; Pfeiffer & Strzelecki, 1990; Gossett, 1985). A study by Lewis (1988) found that measures of family functioning at admission were related to later adjustment. It is clear that young people from dysfunctional families require substantial after-care and support after release from residential care (Curry, 1991; Cornsweet, 1990; Pfeiffer, 1989; Gabel & Shindledecker, 1990; Gossett, 1985). Hence, changes in youngsters produced by residential care often must be accompanied by positive change in the family setting (Curry, 1991; Lewis, 1988).

Researchers have not reached considerable agreement on the value of age, gender, and intelligence as predictors of outcome. For example, Casey and Berman (1985) found that studies which included a greater proportion of male children usually produced smaller treatment effects, while Blotcky et al. (1984) found a slight disadvantage for girls, and a review by Pfeiffer and Strzelecki (1990) found no relationship between sex and outcome.

Weisz et al. (1987) argued that age has a significant effect on outcome, with children faring better than adolescents; however, Pfeiffer and Strzelecki (1990) detected only a weak relationship between age at admission to a psychiatric facility and outcome, and Casey and Berman (1985) found that age did not predict outcome. Kolko (1992), on the other hand, found that older age was predictive of poor short-term outcome. It is important to remember that age at admission to a psychiatric facility, and therefore severity of pathology, may differ as a function of several variables, such as parental anxiety about the hospitalization of their children or ability of schools to handle problem behaviors (Blotcky et al., 1984).

Intelligence is a variable that is often examined in outcome studies. Both Gossett (1985) and Blotcky et al. (1984) found that higher intelligence correlated with greater improvement, while the review by Pfeiffer and Strzelecki (1990) revealed a more modest relationship between intelligence and outcome, and Casey and Berman (1985) found that intellectual functioning was not reliably related to outcome. These inconsistent results may be a function of the fact that tested IQ itself may be affected by psychopathology, and these effects may differ according to severity of disorder. Tested IQ is also correlated with socioeconomic status. Neither of these variables is generally controlled in studies where IQ scores are considered (Blotcky et al., 1984). It may be more informative for studies to employ IQ as an outcome measure as opposed to focusing on IQ as a predictor of outcome (Zimmerman, 1990).

### Correlates of Outcome

Length of hospitalization in a psychiatric facility is a variable that is often considered in studies of inpatient treatment, not as a predictor, but rather as a correlate of outcome. Many children and adolescents improve during inpatient treatment, but an optimal time period for hospitalization has not been clearly established. The operational definition of short-term hospitalization has ranged from 11 days to 89 days, while long-term hospitalization has ranged from 24 days to 179 days. The overlap has meant that what some studies have defined as short-term, others have defined as long-term (Caton, Mayers, & Gralnick, 1990). Therefore, in order to avoid confusion in the interpretation of results from studies of treatment, it is important to consider the researcher's definition of long versus short-term care.

The meta-analysis by Blotcky et al. (1984) found a positive relationship between length of stay and favorable outcome, with most studies suggesting that positive results required hospitalizations of at least 6 months to one year. Pfeiffer and Strzelecki (1990) found a modestly strong positive relationship between longer length of hospitalization and favorable outcome. It appears that, owing to cost cutting by insurance companies, children are increasingly entitled to only brief hospitalizations, regardless of their diagnosis or the severity of their pathology (Caton et al., 1990; Nurcombe, 1989). The results of some studies seem to suggest that shorter hospitalizations may facilitate smoother, less traumatic reintegrations into the family, school and community (Gossett, 1985; Pfeiffer & Strzelecki, 1990). It may be that a rigorous course of post-treatment outpatient care after brief hospitalization can be as effective as traditional, long-term hospitalization in treating psychopathology and preventing rehospitalization (Gunstad & Sherman, 1991; Berman & Austad, 1991).

Ney, Adam, Hanton, and Brindad (1988) found that an important aspect of length of stay is specification, at admission, of exact length of hospitalization. Ney and colleagues argued that knowledge of the exact length of stay helps to concentrate staff effort and foster the involvement of family members, maintaining the children's attachment bonds. Unfortunately, their sample was quite small and therefore not necessarily generalizable. Gunstad and Sherman (1991) similarly argued that discharge planning should begin upon admission to a psychiatric inpatient facility.

Treatment characteristics have not been considered as potential correlates of outcome in most studies and meta-analyses (Blotcky et al., 1984). Representing an exception to this generalization, Casey and Berman (1985) compared the efficacy of different types of treatment, including group versus individual therapy, play versus non-play, and parent-treated versus child-treated. They found no significant differences between these groups. In their comparison of behavioral versus non-behavioral therapies, Weisz et al. (1987) found that behavioral treatments were significantly more effective. It should be noted, however, that studies of behavioral therapies have often employed outcome measures that were very similar to activities occurring during treatment (Blotcky et al., 1984). When these therapy-like measures were removed from the evaluation by Weisz et al. (1987), this difference between behavioral and non-behavioral therapies disappeared. In general, comparisons between different psychotherapeutic techniques have yielded small effect sizes[2] (Kazdin, 1990).

Meta-analysis enables researchers to simultaneously evaluate the findings of a number of studies with different research designs and sample sizes by converting results to a common metric and calculating an overall effect size. Meta-analytic reviews of outcome studies can therefore be instrumental in the identification of common strengths as well as areas of neglect in research (Kazdin, 1993b). Conclusions supported by a combination of many studies may be more reliable than results obtained from a single study.

However, findings of meta-analytic reviews must be interpreted with some degree of caution as a result of the potential repercussions of the process of combining studies. Studies that are reviewed in meta-analyses have often employed different methods of sampling, collecting data, analyzing results, and reporting findings. Differences in outcome that are potentially attributable to differences in sample size, research design, therapeutic technique, and operational definition of improvement may therefore be overlooked (Kazdin, 1993b). Additionally, meta-analysts are often forced to estimate, assume, and infer data that have not been reported, but are nevertheless crucial for the purpose of comparison. Furthermore, meta-analyses generally consider studies that have been published. If there is indeed a publication bias in favor of studies which have obtained significant effects, then meta-analyses have not considered many studies that have failed to produce statistically significant effects.

## SHORTCOMINGS OF CURRENT OUTCOME RESEARCH

Recent evaluations of meta-analytic reviews suggest that meta-analysts may have been overly enthusiastic in their conclusions about the positive effects of treatment (Weisz et al., 1992; Matt, Shadish, Navarro, & Siegle, 1994). An important limitation of many outcome studies that have demonstrated beneficial effects of therapy over no therapy, which has frequently been overlooked, is the fact that the treatment process in the research studies differs significantly from treatment as it is administered in actual clinical practice. Most of the studies evaluated in the aforementioned meta-analyses have included at least one component that makes the study differ from clinical care as it is actually administered. Given important differences between therapy as studied and therapy as actually practiced, positive findings from outcome research may not be generalizable to the treatment that thousands of children and adolescents receive on a daily basis (Weisz et al., 1992; Matt et al., 1994; Kazdin, 1993b).

Several experimental features are commonly found in outcome research. First, many studies use subjects who are volunteers and may therefore represent an entirely different population of children than those who are customarily referred for treatment (Kazdin, 1993b). Children who are recruited for research purposes, for example, may not be as seriously disturbed as those who are clinically referred (Eyberg, 1992). Additionally, samples of subjects are often selected on the basis of similarity of symptoms and dysfunction. Since many children who are diagnosed with one disorder also meet the diagnostic criteria for at least one other disorder, such research samples may be more homogeneous than the general population of youngsters currently receiving psychiatric care (Weisz et al., 1992).

Second, therapists in many studies have been specially trained to administer treatment in accordance with the guidelines of the research design. Therapy sessions are monitored to insure that therapists use only the techniques specified in standardized manuals. Additionally, therapists participating in a research study often carry smaller than average caseloads (Weisz et al., 1992).

These factors may combine to create an artificial therapeutic environment that is optimal for improvement and predesigned to succeed. At the very least, such experimental conditions do not usually constitute mental health services as normally administered. When outcome studies contain laboratory features which make them too dissimilar for comparison with actual therapy as practiced, one may determine only the theoretical efficacy of a particular treatment given the existence of a number of specific conditions (Weisz et al., 1992).

An examination by Weisz et al. (1992) of the clinic-based studies conducted to date indicates that these studies have not yielded the positive results of the laboratory research. In a previous review of studies that contained no laboratory features, Weisz and Weiss (1989) found no significant differences on measures of outcome at the 6 month or one year mark between subjects who completed treatment and those who dropped out after intake (cited in Weisz et al., 1992). Weisz et al. (1992) suggested that poor outcomes may have been related to the fact that most clinic-based studies were conducted decades ago at a "relatively immature stage in the development of therapeutic approaches and standardized assessment of child psychopathology and therapy outcome," but interpreted the results conservatively as evidence that enthusiasm about the significant positive effects produced by psychotherapy may be premature (p. 1584).

Following from the review by Weisz et al. (1992), Matt et al. (1994) endeavored to conduct a comprehensive evaluation of studies in which the treatment closely approximated actual clinical practice. They selected only studies that included subjects referred in the usual fashion and experienced, professional therapists with regular caseloads, conducting therapy in non-university settings. Of the 1,348 studies they reviewed from 23 meta-analyses, only 74 studies from 15 meta-analyses met the conditions for classification as clinically relevant. Matt et al. (1994) calculated weighted average effect sizes for the clinically relevant studies and for the original meta-analyses (which included both laboratory studies and the clinically relevant research). The median effect sizes for the clinically relevant studies and for the original meta-analyses, .48 and .56 respectively, were not significantly different. In all 15 meta-analyses, the 95% confidence intervals for the clinically relevant studies included the median effect sizes for the laboratory studies. Matt and his colleagues admitted that some of the 74 clinically relevant studies may have included the use of manuals or other standardized techniques which are not customarily used in everyday clinical practice. However, they tentatively concluded that these studies provide evidence that psychotherapy as conducted in actual clinical practice is indeed effective. A limitation of Matt and colleagues' meta-analysis for present purposes is that their data consisted mostly of studies of adults.

Whether or not the effectiveness of clinical psychotherapy has been demonstrated by available research, the value of laboratory studies is nevertheless undeniable (Weisz et al., 1992; Matt et al., 1994). Although the positive findings of the meta-analyses may not be generalizable to clinics where treatment occurs on a daily basis, they at least suggest that treatment can be effective if administered in a particular way. The research laboratory may serve as an apt setting for the testing of new treatments, and results obtained may suggest modifications and enhancements to therapy as currently practiced (Weisz et al., 1992). Positive findings regarding innovative treatments or combinations of interventions may be important in that they provide a basis for the introduction of new therapeutic techniques into clinical practice (Weisz et al., 1992; Matt et al., 1994). Of course, the efficacy of these techniques must subsequently be tested in studies of real clinical practice (Matt et al., 1994).

In addition to containing experimental features, many outcome studies also suffer research design flaws that may compromise their generalizability. For example, much outcome research would be more appropriately considered (local) evaluation research. Some studies have focused too specifically on the assessment of the treatment practices of the setting at which the research is being conducted (Cornsweet, 1990). Such studies often have no recognizable research design (Pfeiffer, 1989). All outcome research should have the goal of improved understanding of dysfunction and should therefore be placed in a theoretical framework in which hypotheses may be tested in furtherance of expanding general knowledge about childhood and adolescent disorders (Cornsweet, 1990).

Additionally, many studies employ a test-retest method of measuring effectiveness of treatment, without a no-treatment group or comparison with a sample receiving a different type of treatment (Curry, 1991; Pfeiffer, 1989; Zimmerman, 1990). Studies which lack a no-treatment group fail to control for the potential effects of maturation and the natural course of the disorder (Curry, 1991). Evaluating different treatments without a no-treatment group may also pose significant problems. For example, when two groups receiving different treatments are compared, and the results fail to demonstrate a significant difference between the two, one may conclude only that the treatments had equal effects, but not that both were effective or ineffective (Curry, 1991).

Including no-treatment control groups in experimental designs, although crucial for establishing the basic efficacy of treatment, is often problematic for several reasons. First, it is almost impossible to locate control children who do not differ substantially from treated children on severity of symptoms, level of functioning, family history, socioeconomic background, and other variables which may be predictive of outcome. Second, it is illegal to deny a child services to which he or she is entitled by law. Perhaps most important, it is unethical to withhold mental health services from a child who has been identified as requiring assistance (Bickman, 1992; Weisz et al., 1992; Zimmerman, 1990; Blotcky et al., 1984). Random assignment of disturbed children to treatment and control conditions would necessarily mean that some children would receive no treatment. It has therefore been suggested that control groups could be drawn from children placed on waiting lists for services. However, most waiting lists operate under the principle that the most severe cases should be treated first, thus creating a crucial difference between treated and control subjects (Bickman, 1992; Weisz et al., 1992). Additionally, if a child in the treatment group terminates treatment, a child on the waiting list should not be denied treatment solely to preserve the integrity of the experimental groups. Finally, if a researcher wishes to sufficiently control for effects of maturation and therefore endeavors to follow-up at least one year after termination, control children will necessarily go untreated for over twelve months (Bickman, 1992).

Many outcome studies fail to describe in any detail the setting or the particulars of the treatments administered. Pfeiffer's (1989) review of outcome research found that 34% of the studies made no mention of the type or frequency of treatment, and none considered hospital environment, staff attitudes, or patient-staff relationships. A subsequent review indicated that staff characteristics such as attitudes, level of skill, and interpersonal style do indeed have a significant impact on the success or failure of treatment (Pfeiffer & Strzelecki, 1990). A long term follow-up study of adults who were hospitalized as children found that former patients have stronger memories of paraprofessionals and staff who were involved with them in the accomplishments of specific tasks than of mental health professionals from whom they received psychotherapy (Parham, Reid, & Hamer, 1987). Staff members' perception of a patient as difficult or uncooperative, for example, may disrupt the therapeutic alliance in a way that hinders improvement (Colson et al., 1991).

A large number of studies of child and adolescent mental health services have also provided inadequate information on patient characteristics, such as prior treatment history and diagnostic criteria for inclusion in the study. Pfeiffer (1989) found in a review of 32 outcome studies that 87.5% provided no information about prior treatment, and almost 75% failed to conduct pre-admission evaluations which could later be used as baseline measures. In addition, many studies do not assess patient progress between admission and discharge (Pfeiffer, 1989). Finally, few studies examine the effectiveness of using particular techniques to treat particular dysfunctions. Thus, the empirical basis for matching dysfunction to treatment modality remains fairly weak (Kazdin, 1993a; Blotcky et al., 1984).

## GENERAL OBSTACLES TO CONDUCTING OUTCOME RESEARCH

A major dilemma in the evaluation of favorable outcome for any population is the apparent difficulty in defining "improvement." Besides children, their families, and society as a whole, mental health professionals and third party payers may be counted among those who share a stake in the successful outcome of psychotherapeutic treatment of youngsters. Favorable outcome may of course be defined differently by these various stakeholders. Third party payers, for example, would define successful treatment as that which is least expensive, while parents would define favorable outcome as that which produces a maximal decrease in antisocial or maladaptive behavior of their children, irrespective of cost (Heflinger, 1992). Sometimes, there may be disagreement among stakeholders as to whether a change produced by treatment represents a favorable or unfavorable outcome. For example, a clinician may regard a previously withdrawn and passive adolescent's ability to express normal rebellion toward parents as an indication of positive outcome. The adolescent's parents, for obvious reasons, may not view this behavior in the same positive light (Davis & Frank, 1992). The various stakeholders ultimately would like outcome assessments to measure the particular aspect of improvement that is of concern to them (Heflinger, 1992).

There is clearly a lack of consensus, however, on how improvement should be defined (Berman & Austad, 1991; Pfeiffer & Strzelecki, 1990). Degrees of improvement therefore have varied among studies of child psychotherapy as a function of the operational definition of favorable versus unfavorable outcome (Kazdin, 1990; Vermillion & Pfeiffer, 1993; Pfeiffer & Strzelecki, 1990). One way to conceptualize improvement is in terms of a return to pre-morbid level of positive functioning. However, it is unlikely that positive functioning prior to onset of problems will be well documented in clinical records, so therapists must rely solely on information from the patient or family members regarding pre-morbid functioning (Berman & Austad, 1991).

Increasingly, outcome studies of adult psychotherapy have demonstrated that reduction of symptoms does not always lead to improvement in all areas of functioning, e.g., increased ability to work (Kazdin, 1990). The medical model of "cure" focuses almost exclusively on the absence of symptoms. However, with many disorders, symptoms tend to wax and wane (Pfeiffer, 1989). Therefore, it is equally important to assess positive indications of health when considering outcome and improvement (Heflinger, 1992).

### Content of Outcome Assessment

Measures of outcome vary according to content, source of evaluation, and timing of assessment (Lambert, 1994; Zimmerman, 1990; Weisz et al., 1987; Pfeiffer, 1989). Some studies have operationalized positive versus negative outcome merely in terms of whether a patient returns home or is referred for long-term residential care at discharge from a psychiatric hospital (Gabel & Shindledecker, 1990; Zimmerman, 1990). Similarly, many follow-up studies measure outcome solely on the basis of re-hospitalizations. Although returning home obviously seems to be a more favorable outcome than being referred to a residential facility, decisions about referral can vary widely depending on such factors as the philosophy of the therapist or hospital, and the availability of long term care facilities (Gabel & Shindledecker, 1990). Current scholarly conceptualization of improvement clearly encompasses many factors besides re-hospitalization (e.g., Parham et al., 1987; Kolko, 1992; Klinge et al., 1986; Caton et al., 1990). Implicit in this conceptualization is the understanding that many variables interact to affect outcome, which may be measured along more than one dimension, and be assessed by more than one individual. It is also clear that results obtained from evaluations of outcome, even those that demonstrate a particular treatment has not been effective, may be used to improve upon therapeutic interventions.

Most measures of outcome for children focus on observable behaviors, or quantifiable historical events. For example, outcome has been measured in terms of pre- and post-hospitalization comparisons of school attendance, grade point average, socialization with peers, runaway behavior, illegal activity, and alcohol consumption (Klinge et al., 1986). Improvement has also been measured in terms of physical health and observed adjustment at school and at home (Kazdin, 1990). Although they are readily observed, such objective variables neglect the potential subjective effects of treatment, e.g., improved morale (Cornsweet, 1990). Follow-up studies of adults who were hospitalized as children have measured outcome in terms of marital status, education, employment, perception of self, current relationships, and drug use (Parham et al., 1987). It may be that many outcome measures are interrelated, while others yield independent effects. Therefore, the choice of content of outcome measures may significantly affect the levels of improvement obtained (Kazdin, 1990). For example, in their meta-analytic review of 75 outcome studies, Casey and Berman (1985) observed larger effect sizes for measures of cognitive performance than for measures of self-concept and personality.

### Source of Outcome Assessment

Since outcomes as assessed by individuals with differing perspectives, including parents, therapists, teachers, and children themselves are not highly correlated, the source of the evaluation of outcome may also have a substantial effect on the level of improvement a child is judged to have achieved (Achenbach, 1994; Lachar & Kline, 1994). For example, Weisz et al. (1987) found that observers with no stake in the outcome of treatment reported more change resulting from therapy than did any of the other sources of information about improvement, including parents, teachers, peers and self-reports. In his review of 32 outcome studies, Pfeiffer (1989) found that 68.7% of the outcomes were assessed by only one person. Clearly, this reliance on one source for information about improvement has a substantial–and quite possibly distorting–effect on conclusions about outcome.

Ratings by persons other than the patient may exhibit significant halo effects, as individuals often assign similar ratings to characteristics that are thought to be related even when they have not actually been observed in the child being evaluated. A study of adjustment during residential treatment found that the inter-rater reliability of staff ratings on behavioral rating scales was sometimes as low as .42 (Mordock, 1986). According to Lewis (1988), "whether or not behavior is disturbing is always to some extent a function of the context in which it occurs and the expectations held by other participants in the interaction" (p. 102). Stated another way, children may behave differently depending on the person with whom they are interacting. Children's behavior may also differ substantially from one setting to another (Mordock, 1986; Achenbach, 1994). For example, some children may behave aggressively when in academic settings but have no trouble in peer interactions on the playground. Therefore, it is important that outcomes be evaluated by several persons who play different roles in the lives of the children being assessed (Mordock, 1986).

Parents are commonly asked to evaluate treatment effectiveness with respect to their children. Although children usually spend a considerable amount of their time with their parents, it may be difficult for parents to honestly and objectively assess their children's improvement. For example, a parent who desperately wants a child to be released from the hospital or to avoid having the child re-hospitalized may overstate the child's improvement (Klinge et al., 1986). Most studies of adolescents also include a post-treatment self-rating, while only 43% of child studies include self-ratings (Pfeiffer, 1989). There is some question as to whether children, particularly pre-school aged children, have the cognitive, introspective capabilities to describe their own internal states (Klinge et al., 1986; Eyberg, 1992). Methods for measuring the affective states of children have recently shown great improvement with the development of pictorial instruments (Eyberg, 1992). Outcome measures should certainly include self-assessments for adolescents and, if validity issues can be adequately addressed, measures of subjective well-being ought to be completed by children (Kotsopoulos, Elwood, & Oke, 1989).

### Timing of Outcome Assessment

Some outcome studies evaluate improvements only immediately upon completion of treatment, while others additionally assess progress at one or more follow-up date(s). Researchers have not reached agreement on a standard for timing of follow-up assessments. The time period from termination of treatment to follow-up has varied widely across studies from 6 weeks to over 20 years (Pfeiffer, 1989; Kolko, 1992; Blotcky et al., 1984). In some studies, the mean time period from discharge to follow-up is less than the average length of hospital stay (Klinge et al., 1986).

In their meta-analytic review, Weisz et al. (1987) found that measures of outcome obtained immediately post-treatment were not significantly different from those obtained after an average follow-up period of 6 months. Kolko (1992) did not detect significant differences between outcome assessments at 2, 4, and 6 months post-hospitalization. However, it may be that two month intervals are not long enough to reflect change (Cornsweet, 1990; Lewis, 1988; Kolko, 1992). Improvements observed at discharge from a psychiatric facility, in particular, may represent the favorable effects of removing a child from a dysfunctional environment (Zimmerman, 1990). In order to ensure that variables such as a child's normal maturation or changes in the family environment do not confound interpretation of outcome assessments, Pfeiffer (1989) suggested that follow-up data ought to be collected no earlier than 90 days after discharge and should subsequently be collected at least two additional times: at 6 months post-discharge and at 12-18 months post-discharge.

Assessment of functioning at various times during the follow-up period will inform clinicians about the nature of any gradient of deterioration that becomes evident after treatment has been terminated (Kolko, 1992). Information about follow-up is particularly important in the study of children and adolescents because they are in a continuous state of development, which may independently affect adjustment and the nature and course of a disorder. It is important to ensure that treatments which appear effective in the short run can surpass the effects of developmental change (Kazdin, 1990).

Ideally, improvement should also be assessed at several times during treatment. In their studies of psychotherapy with adults, Howard and his colleagues have demonstrated that improvement progresses through a series of stages (Howard, Lueger, Maling, & Martinovich, 1993). They found that soon after treatment commences, improvement is experienced in terms of an increase in subjective sense of well-being, or restoration of hope on the part of the patient that favorable outcome is possible. This remoralization is necessary, although not sufficient, for transition into the second phase of improvement, in which individuals experience a reduction in symptoms and begin to develop healthier coping skills. Many individuals terminate therapy after symptoms subside and do not experience the final phase of improvement, which is characterized by enhancement of general life-functioning, including the unlearning of maladaptive behaviors. Again, it is necessary, although not sufficient, to experience a reduction of symptoms in order to develop new methods of handling emotions and difficult situations.

This three phase model of improvement has obvious implications for the timing and content of outcome assessments. For example, enhancements in life-functioning, as opposed to reductions in symptoms or improvements in well-being, may not be achieved by an individual who terminates treatment after only a few sessions (Howard et al., 1993).

An important component in the measurement of outcome is the assessment of client satisfaction. Client satisfaction as expressed by both parents and children may be a useful source of information about needed refinements in services (Kotsopoulos et al., 1989). Unfortunately, researchers tend to design their own measures of satisfaction, which makes comparisons across studies more difficult (Heflinger, 1992). Similarly, the most popular instruments used to assess outcome and follow-up are unpublished questionnaires authored by the researcher (Pfeiffer, 1989; Lachar & Kline, 1994). Therefore, measures of outcome differ in a variety of ways. In order to compare the relative success of one treatment versus another, studies must use standardized outcome measures that are validated instruments with known reliabilities (Pfeiffer, 1989; Davis & Frank, 1992; Gabel & Shindledecker, 1990).

Standardization increases generalizability across studies and may serve to refine descriptions of particular dysfunctions. The development of comprehensive, standardized measures of childhood dysfunction has accelerated greatly in the past several years (Kazdin, 1993b). Advancements in the design of measurement tools is one of the most significant accomplishments in the field of therapy outcome research (Eyberg, 1992). For example, the Personality Inventory for Children (PIC) is a parent report measure with a true-false format that may include 131, 280 or 420 items. The PIC assesses areas such as cognitive development, social skills, intellectual achievement, development, somatic symptoms, psychosis and family relations. The Personality Inventory for Youth (PIY) is a self-report measure aimed at children and adolescents aged 9-18. The PIY represents a translation of the first 280 items from the PIC into first-person format. Because the PIY parallels the PIC, administration of both measures enables comparison of child and parent assessments of child functioning. The average correlation between parent and child report is only .25 (Achenbach, McConaughy, & Howell, 1987, cited in Lachar & Kline, 1994). Parents and children differ, for example, in their assessments of child behaviors that are particularly disturbing to adults (e.g., oppositionalism, noncompliance) and problems of which parents are unaware (e.g., substance abuse, sexual activity). Additionally, administration of the PIC to both parents is instrumental in identifying areas of agreement and disagreement (Lachar & Kline, 1994).

Because most items on the PIC and the PIY are written in the present tense, these measures may be administered at several times to assess change attributable to treatment. These are also useful as tools for treatment planning. Since the PIC and the PIY have not yet been used in large numbers of outcome studies, further research is required to test their relative sensitivity to change (Lachar & Kline, 1994).

The Child Behavior Checklist (CBCL) is another omnibus measure of child functioning that has provided the basis for the development of a number of other instruments which may be used to assess childhood dysfunction, including the Child Behavior Checklist for Ages 2-3 (CBCL 2/3), the Direct Observation Form (DOF), the Teacher's Report Form (TRF), and the Youth Self Report (YSR). Like the PIC and the PIY, these measures enable comparisons of ratings from a variety of sources. A cross-informant computer program designed for use with the CBCL and related instruments computes Q correlations to provide a quantitative index of agreement between sources of evaluation (Achenbach, 1994). Again, these instruments may be administered repeatedly in studies of outcome to detect change in functioning (Achenbach, 1994).

Researchers should be cautioned that repeated administrations of the same measure frequently leads to declines in reported problems as a function of regression of deviant scores toward the group mean. However, when assessing the efficacy of several treatments or a treatment and a control, comparison of different group change scores may indicate which treatments were most successful. Researchers should also remember that scores on measures like the TRF and the YSR may be slower to improve than symptom measures, since they include aspects of functioning that take longer to change, such as academic achievement and number of close friends (Achenbach, 1994).

One venerable measure of emotional functioning in children and adolescents has recently been updated. The Devereux Scales of Mental Disorders (DSMD; Naglieri, LeBuffe, & Pfeiffer, 1994a) and the Devereux Behavior Rating Scale-School Form (DBRS; Naglieri, LeBuffe, & Pfeiffer, 1994b) have been in use for nearly three decades and were recently revised and re-normed on a large, national standardization sample. The current version of the DBRS contains 40 items which assess the four areas identified in the federal definition of Serious Emotional Disturbance: interpersonal problems, inappropriate behaviors and feelings, depression, and physical symptoms and fears. The DBRS is usually completed by psychologists, guidance counselors and teachers, but may also be completed by parents. The DSMD may be completed by any adult who has known the child for at least four weeks and because it contains items regarding behaviors such as sleeping and eating habits, is usually filled out by parents. Both the DBRS and the DSMD are available in separate forms for children and adolescents. The 111-item child form and the 110-item adolescent form of the DSMD are based on DSM-IV categories and were designed to identify children and adolescents who are at risk for developing an emotional or behavioral disorder. The Devereux Scales have been proven reliable and valid by a multitude of studies in which they have been included over the past thirty years.

Promising, innovative measures continue to appear. For example, the Behavior Assessment System for Children (BASC) includes scales of positive functioning in addition to psychopathology (Reynolds & Kamphaus, 1992). Ideally, these measures will be able to assist clinicians in treatment planning, monitoring changes over time, and even predicting outcome based on initial case characteristics. In specialized settings, more targeted measures will be more appropriate. The EDI-2 is an example of one such instrument, being designed for use with individuals suffering from anorexia and bulimia. It may also prove more practical to use more targeted instruments to assess the progress and outcome of treatment once a comprehensive assessment using multiscale instruments has pinpointed a youngster's problems. A depressed, suicidal adolescent can be followed with the Reynolds Adolescent Depression Scale (Reynolds, 1987) and the Suicidal Ideation Questionnaire (Reynolds, 1988), while the progress of an adolescent suffering from Attention Deficit Disorder can be assessed with Conners' scales (Conners, 1994).

In the not too distant future, computer adaptive assessment systems will help clinicians make appropriate diagnoses, assign clients to the least expensive appropriate level of care, and monitor treatment more closely, which will provide invaluable information regarding treatment effectiveness. Computer adaptive testing (CAT) allows researchers to measure a construct with greater precision than a fixed-format test while minimizing the number of items administered. In CAT, the computer selects items based on the examinee's responses to previous items. For example, if an alcoholic woman indicated that she was married, the computer would ask her a series of questions about her marriage to determine whether her husband was a source of support or was contributing to the substance abuse. The computer would not pose these questions to patients who reported no significant other in their life. There are commercially published non-psychometric tools such as patient-completed psychological history programs (Giannetti, 1987) and clinician-completed structured interview programs (First, Gibbon, Williams, & Spitzer, 1992) that function in this way. Researchers are working to optimize administration of traditional, fixed-format questionnaires like the MMPI-2 in this fashion (Ben-Porath, Slutske, & Butcher, 1989; Roper, Ben-Porath, & Butcher, 1991).

## SPECIAL CONSIDERATIONS FOR EVALUATING THE EFFECTIVENESS OF TREATMENT OF CHILDREN

Conducting outcome research on the mental health treatment of any population is a complicated process, perhaps in part because mental health treatment–especially psychotherapy–is itself difficult to define, as treatments differ according to theoretical orientation, methods and goals (Kazdin, 1990). In general, the goal of mental health treatment is to decrease symptoms and maladjustment, and increase adaptive and prosocial functioning, although the nature and administration of particular interventions combine with the effects of numerous intervening variables to produce unique outcomes (Kazdin, 1993a).

There are several factors that make it particularly difficult to conduct outcome research with children as opposed to adults. A major difference between the administration of child versus adult mental health services is the fact that children have little, if any, choice regarding the treatment they receive (Kazdin, 1990). Children are almost entirely dependent on adults to meet their basic needs and to define the nature of the environment in which they exist. Therefore, parental dysfunction may particularly affect not only the development of child psychopathology, but also the maintenance of problem behaviors and prospects for successful, post-treatment adjustment (Kazdin, 1993b; Gunstad & Sherman, 1991). Also, child and adolescent disorders are identified and treated in a number of non-mental health service systems, including the educational system, juvenile justice system, health care facilities, and child welfare agencies (Rog, 1992). Concurrent treatment of a child or adolescent in one or more such systems may result in overestimation of the effectiveness of treatment received in a mental health care facility, or may potentially interfere with treatment in significant ways (Bickman, 1992).

Determining whether treatment has been effective in ameliorating childhood psychopathology is also particularly difficult because there is no clear definition of what is "normal" for children and adolescents. Anna Freud (1958) aptly noted that "to be normal during the adolescent period is by itself abnormal" (cited in Powers, Hauler, & Kilner, 1989). The same could be said of childhood. Seemingly "abnormal" behaviors are often quite common and therefore would be more appropriately labeled "normal" during certain developmental phases in childhood and adolescence. For example, simple phobias are fairly common in early childhood, and depressed mood is certainly not uncommon in adolescence (Rutter, 1991).

An important step in defining and measuring childhood dysfunction is greater assessment of normative levels of functioning at various ages, which may serve as a baseline against which to measure pathology (Kazdin, 1993a). Children's sense of mastery and self-confidence depends to some degree on their ability to meet age appropriate expectations regarding their daily living skills, regulation of emotions, and control of behavior. It is only by developing a clearer description of normal behavior at various developmental stages that clinicians will be able to distinguish abnormal from normal facets of behavior and development (Heflinger, 1992).

Another difference between conducting research on children and studying adults is the fact that children are in a state of continuous, and sometimes rapid, development in the social, emotional, physical, cognitive and behavioral domains. Therefore, the presence and progress of dysfunction is confounded by the normal course of development in childhood and adolescence (Kazdin, 1993a; Heflinger, 1992). Much more research is needed regarding the incidence, prevalence and development of dysfunction from childhood through adolescence and into early adulthood to elucidate the onset and course of psychopathology and to disentangle normal developmental issues from psychopathology (Kazdin, 1993a).

The problem of comorbidity is an additional factor that makes evaluating treatment of children and adolescents especially difficult. Roughly one-half of all children and adolescents who are diagnosed with a psychiatric disorder also meet the diagnostic criteria for at least one other disorder (Anderson, Williams, McGee & Silva, 1987). Different problem behaviors may be similar with regard to their utility in achieving particular goals for children, for example, peer acceptance. Therefore, certain disorders, such as substance use and abuse and early sexual activity, for example, commonly occur together (Kazdin, 1993a). Many children with multiple disorders appear to be concurrently affected by biological, familial, and socioeconomic disadvantages (Cornsweet, 1990). Their complex problems will require complex treatments and, consequently, outcome will be hard to characterize succinctly.

Finally, obtaining subjects for research on child and adolescent mental health care may be hampered by parents who fear that participation will increase the likelihood that their child will be stigmatized or labeled.

Proper informed consent should provide an effective solution to this problem (Rog, 1992).

## CONCLUSIONS AND SUGGESTIONS
## FOR FUTURE RESEARCH DIRECTIONS

Whether a treatment has been effective or not, it is important to identify the factors that seem to help or hinder improvement. Treatments that focus exclusively on the child's symptoms may underestimate the effects of other variables that may be contributing to the child's psychopathology and likelihood of responding favorably to treatment. Although studies of outcome are tending toward the inclusion of greater numbers of variables, there are arguably many additional factors to be considered in the evaluation of effectiveness of treatment. Factors that require further examination include: demographic characteristics of the child; family history; treatment combinations; and aspects of the treatment process and environment, including characteristics of the therapist, staff, and facilities (Kazdin, 1993b). Increasing the number of variables in any one study naturally makes it more difficult to evaluate the influence of individual variables. However, studies with few variables risk yielding small or no effects, significantly reducing the chances of replication (Bickman, 1992). Given the time and effort that go into conducting a study of outcome, the advantages of adding variables may outweigh the disadvantages. Once a variable that may be especially predictive of positive outcomes has been identified, it may be subjected to further analysis through experimentation (Kazdin, 1993b).

A variety of non-treatment factors may serve to help or hinder treatment. Therefore, assessment of the general life context in which treatment and recovery are occurring may inform clinicians about the cause for differential outcomes (Moreland et al., 1994). As already noted, it is particularly important to consider parental dysfunction and family life (Blotcky et al., 1984). Child and family characteristics that have received inadequate attention include, but are not limited to: father's presence and involvement in the family; the child's social and interpersonal abilities and perceived alienation from others; attitudes toward parents, rules, and authority figures; and feelings about hospitalization (Pfeiffer & Strzelecki, 1990). In the case of children who spend time in residential facilities, home environmental factors may serve either to bolster or degrade gains made during residential treatment (Lewis, 1988). Unless family pathology and dysfunction are addressed in treatment, the symptoms that prompted admission of a child or adolescent to a hospital or residential care facility may reappear upon discharge (Mordock, 1986).

The extent of comorbidity of disorders in childhood and adolescence highlights the need for further research on the effectiveness of combinations of treatment techniques. Although there are more than 230 different therapeutic techniques currently used to treat children and adolescents (Kazdin, 1993a), approximately one-half of all outcome studies conducted to date have assessed cognitive behavioral and behavior modification techniques (Kazdin, 1993b). There is also a need for research on the effectiveness of particular treatments relative to controls–either no treatment or other treatments (Kazdin, 1993b). Kazdin (1990) suggested that, as those studying adults have done, researchers should dispense with the question of whether treatment of children and adolescents works in favor of the more specific question: "What treatment, by whom, is most effective for this individual with that specific problem, under which set of circumstances" (p. 30).

Recent meta-analyses highlight the need for research designed to more clearly define improvement through standardization of outcome measures. Although several excellent measures of child functioning have recently been developed, researchers continue to use their own measures, precluding generalization. Another important goal of researchers should be the use of standardized measures of the child's baseline condition against which outcome may be assessed. Despite standards for diagnoses based on presenting symptoms, different facilities may evaluate a patient differently as a function of ideological, socioeconomic, clinical, or historical factors (Cornsweet, 1990).

Few research studies have focused on the differential effects of outpatient versus inpatient care. Even fewer studies have compared the efficacy of hospitalization versus treatment in a residential facility. Owing to a paucity of studies, some recent meta-analyses have either combined inpatient with outpatient studies (e.g., Casey & Berman, 1985), or combined studies of residential and hospital treatment (e.g., Blotcky et al., 1984). Comparisons of residential treatment and hospital treatment seem particularly important since the nature of the population of children and adolescents in hospitals has changed as a result of the increasing numbers of private residential programs and the restrictions on coverage imposed by health care providers. The patients in hospitals are more chronically disturbed, harder to manage, and more likely to be diagnosed as having serious antisocial problems. Although residential care facilities have not been studied extensively, it seems that the patients treated are less severely disturbed (Cornsweet, 1990). It must be recognized, however, that these comparisons will provide only a coarse first approximation. The characteristics of patients at two "residential facilities" can differ widely, depending on the geographic location, differential referral practices, and orientation or specialty of the facility (Gabel & Shindledecker, 1990).

Another potential area for research is whether childhood and adolescence are different enough from each other to warrant separate consideration in outcome research (Kazdin, 1993a). Weisz et al. (1987) found, in their meta-analytic review of 108 outcome studies, that psychotherapy was significantly more effective for children than for adolescents. They suggested that this finding may be explained by the fact that adolescents are more cognitively complex, have more entrenched problems, and tend to be more resistive of adult authority, which makes them more resistant to change. However, Weisz et al. also pointed out that, theoretically, adolescents ought to be more receptive than children to therapeutic intervention, given that they are better able to understand the purpose of therapy and the psychological determinants of behavior.

A major criticism of outcome studies conducted to date is the pervasive use of simple statistical procedures such as t-tests, chi-square and correlational analyses, as opposed to more powerful and sophisticated techniques (Pfeiffer & Strzelecki, 1990). Outcome assessments must begin to include multivariate statistical models capable of performing more complex comparisons with greater power (Blotcky et al., 1984). Multiple regression, for example, provides information about how much variation in an outcome measure may be explained by a number of predictor variables (Pfeiffer, 1989).

Finally, a major priority for research must be bridging the gap between clinical practice and experimental work by conducting studies in the settings in which treatment is actually administered (Kazdin, 1990). Clinical work with children often occurs under unpredictable, uncontrolled circumstances (Blotcky et al., 1984) However, greater collaboration between researchers and practicing clinicians will enable children and adolescents to benefit from their collective expertise (Weisz et al., 1992). Unfortunately, health care administrators are often wary of conducting research that they believe will be costly and disruptive to normal delivery of services. Clinicians resist participation in outcome studies because research inevitably involves additional paperwork, which requires commitment of additional time. Managed health care systems, which are already subject to utilization review and quality control seem well-suited to integrate research as a routine part of the administration of care (Berman & Austad, 1991). Collecting outcome data as part of continuous quality improvement is a cost-effective method of evaluating the effectiveness of a specific program while increasing general knowledge about the treatment of youngsters (Vermillion & Pfeiffer, 1993).

In summary, treatment designed specifically for children has advanced considerably since the custodial era of mental health care for disturbed youngsters. However, treatment design and implementation requires further refinement, and operationalization of outcomes must be clearer. All individuals who conduct outcome research would agree that it requires an incredible amount of time, energy, and resources (Parham et al., 1987; Kazdin, 1990). However, the benefits of curtailing psychopathology in children and adolescents extends from the troubled youngsters themselves to families, communities, and society as a whole.

## NOTES

1. Meta-analysis refers to a method of evaluating several studies simultaneously through quantification of results in a way that allows calculation of an overall effect size (see below).
2. Effect size is a quantification of the degree of change produced by a treatment.

## REFERENCES

Achenbach, T. M. (1994). Child behavior checklist and related instruments. In M.E. Maruish (Ed.), *The use of psychological testing for treatment planning and outcome assessment* (pp. 517-549). Hillsdale, NJ: Erlbaum.

Ben-Porath, Y. S., Slutske, W. S., & Butcher, J. N. (1989). A real-data simulation of computerized adaptive administration of the MMPI. *Psychological Assessment, 1*, 18-22.

Berman, W. H., & Austad, C. S. (1991). Managed mental health care: Current status and future directions. In C. S. Austad & W. H. Berman (Eds.), *Psychotherapy in managed health care* (pp. 264-278). Washington, DC: American Psychological Association.

Bickman, L. (1992). Designing outcome evaluations for children's mental health services: Improving internal validity. *New Directions for Program Evaluation, 54*, 57-68.

Blotcky, M. J., Dimperio, T. L., & Gossett, J. T. (1984). Follow-up of children treated in psychiatric hospitals: A review of studies. *American Journal of Psychiatry, 141*, 1499-1507.

Casey, R. J., & Berman, J. S. (1985). The outcome of psychotherapy with children. *Psychological Bulletin, 98*, 388-400.

Caton, C. L. M., Mayers, L., & Gralnick, A. (1990). The long-term hospital treatment of the young chronic patient: Follow-up findings. *The Psychiatric Hospital, 21*, 25-30.

Colson, D. B., Cornsweet, C., Murphy, T., O'Malley, F., Hyland, P. S., McParland, M., & Coyne, L. (1991). Perceived treatment difficulty and therapeutic alliance on an adolescent psychiatric hospital unit. *American Journal of Orthopsychiatry, 61,* 221-229.

Conners, C. K. (1994). Conners Rating Scales. In M.E. Maruish (Ed.), *The use of psychological testing for treatment planning and outcome assessment* (pp. 550-578). Hillsdale, NJ: Erlbaum.

Cornsweet, C. (1990). A review of research on hospital treatment of children and adolescents. *Bulletin of the Menninger Clinic, 54,* 64-77.

Crits-Christoph, P. (1992). The efficacy of brief dynamic psychotherapy: A meta-analysis. *American Journal of Psychiatry, 149,* 151-158.

Curry, J. F. (1991). Outcome research on residential treatment: Implications and suggested directions. *American Journal of Orthopsychiatry, 61,* 348-357.

Davis, K. E., & Frank, R. G. (1992). Integrating costs and outcomes. *New Directions for Program Evaluation, 54,* 69-84.

Day, D. M., Pal, A., & Goldberg, K. (1994). Assessing the post-residential functioning of latency-aged conduct disordered children. *Residential Treatment for Children & Youth, 11,* 45-61.

Eyberg, S. M. (1992). Assessing therapy outcome with preschool children: Progress and problems. *Journal of Clinical Child Psychology, 21,* 306-311.

First, M. B., Gibbon, M., Williams, J. B. W., & Spitzer, R. L. (1992). *AutoSCID I.* [computer program]. Toronto: Multi-Health Systems.

Gabel, S., & Shindledecker, R. (1990). Parental substance abuse and suspected child abuse/maltreatment predict outcome in children's inpatient treatment. *Journal of American Academy of Child and Adolescent Psychiatry, 29,* 919-924.

Giannetti, R. A. (1987). The GOLPH psychosocial history: Response-contingent data acquisition and reporting. In J. N. Butcher (Ed.), *Computerized psychological assessment: A practitioner's guide* (pp. 124-144). New York: Basic Books.

Gossett, J. T. (1985). Psychiatric hospital follow-up study: Current findings and future directions. *Psychiatric Annals, 15,* 596-601.

Gunstad, M., & Sherman, C. F. (1991). A model of adolescent inpatient short-term treatment. In C. S. Austad & W. H. Berman (Eds.), *Psychotherapy in managed health care* (pp. 126-137). Washington, DC: American Psychological Association.

Heflinger, C. A. (1992). Client-level outcomes of mental health services for children and adolescents. *New Directions for Program Evaluation, 54,* 31-46.

Howard, K. I., Lueger, R. J., Maling, M. S., & Martinovich, Z. (1993). A phase model of psychotherapy outcome: Causal mediation of change. *Journal of Consulting and Clinical Psychology, 61,* 678-685.

Kazdin, A. E. (1990). Psychotherapy for children and adolescents. *Annual Review of Psychology, 41,* 21-54.

Kazdin, A. E. (1993a). Adolescent mental health: Prevention and treatment programs. *American Psychologist, 48,* 127-141.

Kazdin, A. E. (1993b). Psychotherapy for children and adolescents. *American Psychologist, 48,* 644-657.

Klinge, V., Piggott, L., Knitter, E., & O'Donnell, A. (1986). A follow-up study of psychiatrically hospitalized adolescents. *Adolescents, 21,* 697-701.

Kolko, D. J. (1992). Short-term follow-up of child psychiatric hospitalization: Clinical description, predictors, and correlates. *Journal of American Academy of Child and Adolescent Psychiatry, 31,* 719-727.

Kotsopoulos, S., Elwood, S., & Oke, L. (1989). Parent satisfaction in a child psychiatric service. *Canadian Journal of Psychiatry, 34,* 530-533.

Lachar, D., & Kline, R. B. (1994). Personality inventory for children and personality inventory for youth. In M. E. Maruish (Ed.), *The use of psychological testing for treatment planning and outcome assessment* (pp. 479-516). Hillsdale, NJ: Erlbaum.

Lambert, M. J. (1994). Use of psychological tests for outcome assessment. In M. E. Maruish (Ed.), *The use of psychological testing for treatment planning and outcome assessment* (pp. 75-97). Hillsdale, NJ: Erlbaum.

Lewis, W. W. (1988). The role of ecological variables in residential treatment. *Behavioral Disorders, 13,* 98-107.

Matt, G. E., Shadish, W. R., Jr., Navarro, A. M., & Siegle, G. (1994, November). *Generalizing from the research lab to clinical practice: A reanalysis of psychotherapy meta-analyses.* Paper presented at the American Evaluation Association Annual Meeting, Boston, MA.

Mordock, J. B. (1986). The inadequacy of formal measures of child adjustment during residential treatment. *Residential Treatment for Children & Youth, 4,* 55-73.

Moreland, K. L., Fowler, R. D., & Honaker, L. M. (1994). Future directions in the use of psychological assessment for treatment planning and outcome assessment: Predictions and recommendations. In M. E. Maruish (Ed.), *The use of psychological testing for treatment planning and outcome assessment* (pp. 581-602). Hillsdale, NJ: Erlbaum.

Naglieri, J. A., LeBuffe, P. A., & Pfeiffer, S. I. (1994a). *Devereux Scales of Mental Disorders manual.* San Antonio, TX: The Psychological Corporation.

Naglieri, J. A., LeBuffe, P. A., & Pfeiffer, S. I. (1994b). *Devereux Behavior Rating Scale-School Form manual.* San Antonio, TX: The Psychological Corporation.

Ney, P. G., Adam, R. R., Hanton, B. R., & Brindad, E. S. (1988). The effectiveness of a child psychiatric unit: A follow-up study. *Canadian Journal of Psychiatry, 33,* 793-799.

Nurcombe, B. (1989). Goal-directed treatment planning and the principles of brief hospitalization. *Journal of American Academy of Child and Adolescent Psychiatry, 28,* 26-30.

Parham, C., Reid, S., & Hamer, R. M. (1987). A long-range follow-up study of former inpatients at a children's psychiatric hospital. *Child Psychiatry and Human Development, 17,* 199-209.

Pfeiffer, S. I. (1989). Follow-up of children and adolescents treated in psychiatric facilities: A methodology review. *The Psychiatric Hospital, 20,* 15-20.

Pfeiffer, S. I., & Strzelecki, S. C. (1990). Inpatient psychiatric treatment of children and adolescents: A review of outcome studies. *Journal of American Academy of Child and Adolescent Psychiatry, 29,* 847-853.

Powers, S. I., Hauser, S. T., & Kilner, L. A. (1989). Adolescent mental health. *American Psychologist, 44,* 200-208.

Reynolds, C. R., & Kamphaus, R. W. (1992). *BASC (Behavior Assessment System for Children) manual.* Circle Pines, MN: American Guidance Service.

Reynolds, W. M. (1987). *Reynolds Adolescent Depression Scale professional manual.* Odessa, FL: Psychological Assessment Resources.

Reynolds, W. M. (1988). *Suicidal Ideation Questionnaire professional manual.* Odessa, FL: Psychological Assessment Resources.

Rog, D. J. (1992). Child and adolescent mental health services: Evaluation challenges. *New Directions for Program Evaluation, 54,* 5-16.

Roper, B. L., Ben-Porath, Y. S., & Butcher, J. N. (1991). Comparability of computerized adaptive and conventional testing with the MMPI-2. *Journal of Personality Assessment, 57,* 278-290.

Rutter, M. (1991). Age changes in depressive disorders: Some developmental considerations. In J. Garber & K. Dodge (Eds.), *The development of emotion regulation and dysregulation* (pp. 273-300). Cambridge, England: Cambridge University Press.

Shadish, W. R., Montgomery, L. M., Wilson, P., Wilson, M. R., Bright, I., & Okwumabua, T. (1993). Effects of family and marital psychotherapies: A meta-analysis. *Journal of Consulting and Clinical Psychology, 61,* 992-1002.

Vermillion, J. M., & Pfeiffer, S. I. (1993). Treatment outcome and continuous quality improvement: Two aspects of program evaluation. *The Psychiatric Hospital, 24,* 9-14.

Weisz, J. R., Weiss, B., Alicke, M. D., & Klotz, M. L. (1987). Effectiveness of psychotherapy with children and adolescents: A meta-analysis for clinicians. *Journal of Consulting and Clinical Psychology, 55,* 542-549.

Weisz, J. R., Weiss, B., & Bononberg, G. R. (1992). The lab versus the clinic: Effects of child and adolescent psychotherapy. *American Psychologist, 47,* 1578-1585.

Yokley, J. M., Coleman, D. J., & Yates, B. T. (1990). Cost effectiveness of three child mental health assessment methods: Computer assisted assessment is effective and inexpensive. *Journal of Mental Health Administration, 17,* 99-107.

Zimmerman, D. P. (1990). Notes on the history of adolescent inpatient and residential treatment. *Adolescence, 15,* 9-38.

# Criteria for Selecting Instruments to Assess Treatment Outcomes

Rex S. Green, PhD
Frederick L. Newman, PhD

**SUMMARY.** A process is proposed for identifying optimal outcome assessment instruments for residential studies, and an example is provided of the application of this process. The five steps of the process are: (1) decide what to measure, (2) identify unwanted effects to measure, (3) develop an assessment plan that covers all areas of assessment, (4) tally the candidate assessment instruments by area, and (5) evaluate rival instruments within an area by applying the ideal outcome measure criteria (Newman & Ciarlo, 1994). Because the success of empirical studies depends on the proper selection of assessment instruments, it is recommended that this process be followed whenever significant changes in an assessment battery are planned. *[Article copies available from The Haworth Document Delivery Service: 1-800-342-9678. E-mail address: getinfo@haworth.com]*

One of the more demanding tasks in designing field studies of the effectiveness of residential services is the selection of appropriate outcome assessment tools. What should be measured? Are there assessment instru-

---

Rex S. Green is a consultant in private practice in Cupertino, CA. Frederick L. Newman is affiliated with Florida International University.

Preparation of this article was supported in part by a Center for Mental Health Services Grant R18-MH49157 to Frederick L. Newman.

Dr. Green may be written at 20990 Valley Green Drive #710, Cupertino, CA 95014.

[Haworth co-indexing entry note]: "Criteria for Selecting Instruments to Assess Treatment Outcomes." Green, Rex S., and Frederick L. Newman. Co-published simultaneously in *Residential Treatment for Children & Youth* (The Haworth Press, Inc.) Vol. 13, No. 4, 1996, pp. 29-48; and: *Outcome Assessment in Residential Treatment* (ed: Steven I. Pfeiffer) The Haworth Press, Inc., 1996, pp. 29-48. Single or multiple copies of this article are available from The Haworth Document Delivery Service [1-800-342-9678, 9:00 a.m. - 5:00 p.m. (EST). E-mail address: getinfo@haworth.com].

© 1996 by The Haworth Press, Inc. All rights reserved.

ments available? What works? Where can you find more in-depth information about the assessment? Will it work for the population under study? Must staff be trained to administer it? What is the likely total cost of obtaining and administering the instrument? Are there other assessments that work nearly as well for a smaller total cost, including acquisition, duplication, training, administration, data storage, scoring, and utilization of results?

The purpose of this report is to recommend a structure for the task of selecting treatment outcome assessment instruments. The recommended structure has five steps. Although the steps should be performed in order, they may be performed at any time in conjunction with the other tasks of designing a study. The five steps are:

1. Deciding what to measure, i.e., the concept or construct.
2. Identifying the unintended/unwanted effects.
3. Organizing an assessment plan to address all constructs.
4. Identifying the assessment instruments that fit the plan.
5. Evaluating rival instruments and selecting appropriately.

A reminder to fully address the first two steps seems in order, since our tendency is to assume we already know what to measure. True, the first step may add only a little information for persons familiar with the treatment theories and constructs specified by the theories. However, rethinking the theoretical connections may yield new insights. Also, seeking recently developed information from the literature may yield a surprise or two. Step two can be time-consuming, not to mention challenging. The most likely payoffs are the development of a richer theoretical model and the identification of causal relations that confound or suppress the effects of interest. Each step is described below in relation to the literature. Also, a hypothetical example is presented to illustrate how the steps are applied.

### *STEP ONE–WHAT TO MEASURE*

When conducting applied research on existing treatments in actual settings, it is just as important to specify the treatment theory as when conducting controlled trials in laboratory settings. Lipsey (1993) likens this step to opening the black box of service delivery, so that the connections between the inputs, treatment processes, and treatment outcomes become clear. Unless the treatment process connections are elucidated, at best a hit-and-miss approach follows for connecting the treatment outcomes to inputs. When little or no effect is captured by the treatment outcome assessments, it is difficult to determine whether the inputs were insufficient, the treatment processes were weakly implemented or ineffectual, or the assessments themselves were inappropriate or inaccurate.

Lipsey provides several specific suggestions for replacing the blackbox. One suggestion is to diagram the connections and articulate what program personnel think must occur during treatment, as in Figure 1. Arrows can be drawn from known inputs to suspected processes, thence to likely outcomes. The plausibility of the diagrammed connections can be tested on other investigators, program administrators, and program staff before deciding which constructs to measure. One additional benefit of being more explicit about the treatment processes is the discovery of intermediate outcomes. Some treatment effects may show up sooner, others later. The intermediate outcomes can be assessed, too, assuming some consideration is paid to when to apply the assessment instruments.

Two additional sources of constructs, or statements of what to assess such as level of aggressive behavior, derive from program goals and the values of program stakeholders. Once the treatment theory is developed, there is likely to be considerable overlap between the theoretical constructs of treatment outcomes and the stated goals of a residential program. Reasoning in reverse, by formalizing the program's goals, some of the same constructs can be identified as by articulating the treatment theory. The specification of behavioral objectives as program goals is cited by House (1980) as one of the early approaches to evaluating social programs. Suchman (1967) focused primarily on this approach in his pioneering work on program evaluation. By specifying the goals of the residential treatment program and diagraming the linkages between service activities and goals, discrepancies between what ought to occur (based on theory) and what is desired (behavioral objectives) can be highlighted. Under some circumstances, it may be desirable to include treatment outcome assessments representing both views.

The other source of constructs stems from the values stakeholders in a program possess. Some of the stakeholders for a residential treatment program include the program director, program staff, residents under treatment, parents of the residents, and administrators within agencies that provide funding for the program. "Stakeholder analysis" (Ackoff, 1975) was developed to clarify these values and seek a balance of conflicting values or claims relating to what a treatment program should accomplish. Surveys of stakeholder values (Lawrence & Cook, 1982) can be designed and conducted to gain a broader understanding of the treatment outcomes that should be measured.

FIGURE 1. Two models of the structure, process, and outcomes of group counseling for adolescent males with conduct disorder; the group counseling model is represented in the overall study model as dosage—number of meetings missed and number of dyadic exchanges.

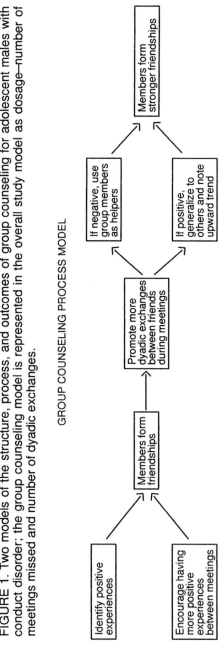

GROUP COUNSELING PROCESS MODEL

# STRUCTURE - PROCESS - OUTCOME STUDY MODEL

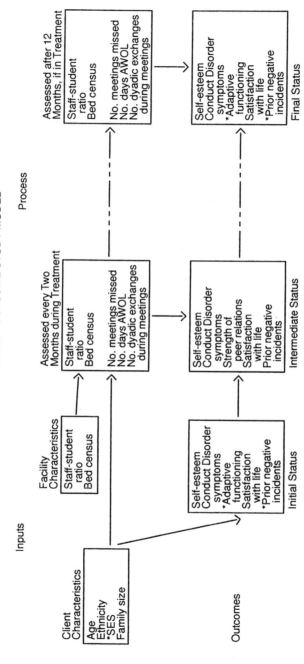

* Refers to assessments provided by the family of a client.

33

## STEP TWO–UNINTENDED/UNWANTED EFFECTS

Far more occurs as a result of delivering residential treatments than is specified by the treatment theory or program goals. The relevance of some of the "unintended effects" of treatment to the experience of being a patient are notable. Other unintended effects impact program staff and have the potential to interact with treatment processes. It is likely that most of the unintended effects will be unwanted outcomes. Thus, a fast start on developing the list of unintended effects is to answer the question, "What might happen as a result of providing this treatment that will prevent the program from achieving its goals?" Perhaps of greater interest, but more difficult to discern, are the positive unintended effects. Sherrill (1984) develops several approaches to identifying unintended effects and argues for measuring the associated outcomes. Some of the sources he mentions include: further elaboration of the treatment theory to surface more of the effects produced, applying systems analysis to the operation of the residential program, identifying the opponents of the treatment program and what their concerns are, reviewing the regulations governing the establishment and operation of the program, and soliciting input from an advisory board to the program. Still other sources are: a review of the literature covering the treatment and what was noted as an unintended result, interviewing program staff and residents about the lesser known developments, and reviewing local program policies for potential problems that may impact on treatment outcomes. The search for unintended effects may be one of the keys to improving treatment outcome results for patients, either by documenting positive unintended effects or gaining more control over the negative ones, once their impact is better understood.

## STEP THREE–AN ASSESSMENT PLAN

As the constructs accumulate from applying the first two steps, it will become clear that the study design should include multiple measures. Because the information about the status of a resident may derive from more than one source, for example, the resident and a member of the staff, it may also be necessary to select multiple measures for the same construct. If there is interest in generalizing from the results across settings, then two or more contexts may be sampled to assess the same construct, such as a school setting in addition to the treatment facility.

Rosenblatt and Attkisson (1993) describe a model for distinguishing these various possibilities. They recommend that mental health services research studies of more severely ill persons consider reporting on the outcomes across four domains: clinical status, functional status, life satisfaction, and public safety. They cite five types of respondents who may serve as sources of data, including the client, family members, social acquaintances, clinical staff, or scientists who conduct research. The data may arise within one or more of four social contexts, the client as an individual, family life, work or school settings, and all other connections to the community. Their model suggests a way to develop a treatment outcome assessment plan for deciding which assessment instruments to include in a study. Once the list of constructs is formed, the constructs can be entered into the cells of a table depicting as many of the cells from the Rosenblatt and Attkisson model as are needed to summarize treatment outcomes for the study. The creation of this table and the manipulation of its rows and columns can be facilitated by utilizing a computerized spreadsheet program.

## STEP FOUR–INSTRUMENTS THAT FIT THE PLAN

There are numerous sources of information about treatment outcome assessments for children and youth to review for locating the instruments (Hammill et al., 1992; Heflinger, 1992; Hodges, 1992; Johnson et al., 1971; Johnson, 1976; Maruish, 1994, National Institute of Mental Health, 1983; National Institute of Mental Health, 1984; Pfeiffer et al., 1992). Another way to obtain information about treatment outcome assessment involves three steps. First, review recently published articles that may cite instruments containing measures of the constructs in your assessment plan. Second, obtain a copy of the article(s) and the instrument. In some instances, developers turn their products over to a software distributor. Many of the companies that market tests and other types of assessment instruments are listed in *Tests* (Sweetland & Keyser, 1991) or, if the instrument is computerized, in *Psychware Sourcebook* (Krug, 1987). If an article cites a government publication, order a free copy by writing or calling either the specific department or U.S. Government Publications. Third, search the Social Science Index that covers recent citations of earlier articles. Further information about the application of a particular instrument may be available from the author of a recently published article.

Some measures are not written instruments but ways of obtaining the needed information. Nelson (1981) reviews the advantages of several of these methods, including diaries, observational counts, archival records, physiological response measures, and behavioral by-products. For further information on unobtrusive measures, refer to Webb, Campbell, Schwartz and Sechrest (1970).

As assessment instruments are located, the constructs measured by the scales contained in the instrument are compared to the constructs listed in the assessment plan. When there is a match, the construct listed in the plan can be annotated with a code for the assessment instrument; subsequent sortings of the list on this field will pull all constructs together that a single instrument measures. By returning the table to the original ordering, the variety of instruments that supply scales for one construct can again be examined.

With a little persistence in tracking down the assessments needed, it is likely that more than one assessment instrument will contribute scales to some of the cells in the assessment plan. While there is no need to include every assessment instrument mentioned in the above sources, your assessment plan should contain some overlapping coverage of the constructs listed. Once numerous cells in your assessment plan contain two or more similar scales, then it is time to apply the next step–picking the best instrument(s) for application during the study.

## STEP FIVE–EVALUATING RIVAL INSTRUMENTS

Decisions between assessment instruments must be made, when two or more measures of the same construct are noted within a cell of the assessment plan. The application of the following 11 criteria (Newman & Ciarlo, 1994) will increase one's confidence in selecting more appropriate instruments. Two levels of comparisons are required. At the lower level, similar scales within each cell of the assessment plan are compared using the 11 criteria. At the higher level, some form of scoring each assessment instrument based on the results of the comparisons at the lower level will simplify the task of selecting among treatment outcome assessment instruments. However, there may be instances in which you lack the time to administer several entire instruments. In this situation, consider whether distinct scales can be extracted from larger assessment instruments. If this alternative proves appealing, then some combination of the higher scoring scales may be formed as a questionnaire to be administered during your study.

Here are a few tips on ways of simplifying the process of comparing similar scales across the 11 criteria. When information is obtained that pertains to the entire assessment instrument, but not to individual scales contained in the instrument, consider whether this information does apply to every scale. If so, use the same information when comparing any scale contained in that instrument to another scale. When the scales within an instrument possess similar characteristics, for example, when the response categories are the same for all questions, it may be possible to evaluate the scales within the instrument similarly on several of the criteria. Consider soliciting the opinions of the staff who will administer the measures. Have them rate example scales from several competing instruments on some, if not all, of the 11 criteria. Combine these results with other information you obtain about the measures before choosing among scales, then among instruments.

*Criterion 1–Relevance to Target Group.* The scale that contains response choices relating to persons in the target group is preferred to one that appears difficult to apply. For example, one scale has been tested on persons of the same age and ethnicity that will be studied and indications of high reliability and validity were noted. This scale is preferred to one that has not been applied to the same target group before, or when it was, did not demonstrate good psychometric properties.

*Criterion 2–Simple, Teachable Methods.* Some scales are difficult to understand and apply, while others appear straightforward. Scales that are more readily grasped by whoever applies them are preferred. When clear instructions, manuals, and training programs are made available, some scales that require more effort to grasp may still perform well. Simple-appearing scales may not be easy to apply, because they lack adequate guidelines for the category choices. When judging this criterion, it is advisable to actually try to pilot test the scales being compared.

*Criterion 3–Measures with Objective Referents.* Scales with category anchors covering observable behaviors are preferred. Scales with brief adjectival anchors may be interpreted differently by those who apply the scale. Scales with no anchoring descriptions are the least preferred. Scales with referents requiring special knowledge or training to interpret, should be investigated before concluding that they will perform well in your setting.

*Criterion 4–Use of Multiple Respondents.* There is some appeal to utilizing a scale for which the same or a related version may be applied by a different type of respondent, or source of data. The comparisons of views across respondents may be facilitated, or the process of combining reports from different respondents may be easier to justify.

*Criterion 5–Process-Identifying Measures.* To the extent that the content of a measure reflects the treatment processes thought to cause better outcomes, or the scale scores seem related to process variables, then higher outcome scores might be interpreted as a sign the treatment is more effective. Because the application of this criterion is more complex and the debate continues regarding its importance, its use remains somewhat tentative.

*Criterion 6–Psychometric Strengths.* The folding of several psychometric criteria into this one criterion makes its application more complex. The several sub-criteria to be considered include: one or more forms of reliability, all types of validity, sensitivity to treatment-related change, and non-reactivity to user biases and situational factors. Applying this criterion requires locating articles covering the performance of the scale and/or conducting a pilot test of the scale's application within the treatment setting. The sub-criteria are not necessarily equally important. For studies of treatment effectiveness, Stewart and Archbold (1992, 1993) recommend emphasizing sensitivity to change. In their view content validity should be emphasized over construct validity and increasing the number of items or raters to improve reliability is the most effective way to increase the power of the measure to detect group differences, thereby raising the power of the study design. Consider, too, that the quality of the service is probably related to the reliability of the scale. If different members of the clinical team use a scale differently, then it will perform less reliably. Probably, they see the consumer in different ways. These differences will likely lead to discontinuities of care and thereby reduce the quality of care. Newman and associates (Newman, Kopta, McGovern, Howard, & McNeilly, 1988; Newman, Fitt, and Heverly, 1987) have demonstrated how vulnerable rating scales are to biasing influences. When comparing rating scales with each other, or other measures, the likelihood of bias arising should be considered, along with what steps may be needed to reduce the occurrence of biased ratings.

*Criterion 7–Low Cost.* Provided all the costs of implementing a particular scale are considered, the lower costing scale is preferred. After estimating the more obvious costs, acquisition, administration, coding, and storage of data, other less obvious costs should be examined. What will be the cost of training and retraining research staff to apply the scale? These costs might include a pilot reliability/validity study. How likely is it that the scale wording will need revision sometime during the study? If the scoring is complicated, how much more will it cost to hire the expertise to set up a computerized scoring program? Is the scale prone to errorful application, leading to missing data or revised analyses? Obviously, there are many ways of considering the total cost; spending time considering different possibilities may well save precious research resources.

*Criterion 8–Understanding by Nonprofessional Audiences.* This criterion is the first of four concerning the utility of the scores beyond the immediate needs of the research study. Depending on the circumstances surrounding the conduct of the study, these criteria will assume greater or lesser importance. It is unlikely they will be of greater importance than the preceding seven criteria, since the first seven criteria relate more directly to the conduct of a research study. As with the next criterion, it is advisable to solicit input from an audience to which the scores will be presented before concluding how understandable they are. Also, consider whether the scores can be relabeled to improve their understandability.

*Criterion 9–Easy Feedback and Uncomplicated Interpretation.* With a dash of creativity, most scales can be transformed so their scores are more readily interpreted. If too much creativity appears to be needed, then the scale most difficult to transform may be less preferred. Downplaying the relative importance of these two criteria is not meant to slight the importance of taking these steps to inform all stakeholders about program results. However, different audiences react more positively to different styles of presentation. The more stakeholder groups there are, the greater the need to pursue different transformations of the scores to suit each group.

*Criterion 10–Usefulness in Clinical Services.* There is an advantage to considering how useful a scale might be to the clinical staff of the treatment facility. If the staff are to apply the scale as part of a study, they are more likely to provide accurate reports when applying a scale that they find useful in assessing service need, style or length of treatment, likelihood of reimbursement, or responsiveness to treatment. In other words, will staff see the scale as relevant to their concerns?

*Criterion 11–Compatibility with Clinical Theories and Practices.* Assuming that staff of the treatment facility possess diverse experiences and professional orientations, and they are required to apply a scale, that scale which is least steeped in one clinical theory is to be preferred. For surely, those staff members who are most comfortable with the theory behind a scale will apply the scale differently from those who are not.

## CHOOSING INSTRUMENTS FOR A NEW STUDY

The application of the five steps and eleven criteria to select treatment outcome assessments becomes clearer when actually designing a study of treatment effectiveness. The following hypothetical example simulates the design of a study to obtain federal funding for comparing two psychotherapy treatments provided by a chain of 10 adolescent group homes. Many of the choices made to illustrate the application of the five steps deserve more debate; each choice might have been made in other ways, given more information. While it is more desirable to take additional time and gather more complete information, for the sake of this example, it is assumed that there was not time to be more thorough.

The Family Way chain of 10 group homes for involuntarily placed adolescent males with a conduct disorder decided to apply for a grant to revise their psychotherapeutic services. Typically, each resident is treated for 9 to 12 months, then placed back in the community. An intensive form of three times per week group counseling was recently written up as being effective for this diagnostic group. Based on the findings of Howard et al. (1993), the focus of the counseling concentrates on building feelings of well-being first, followed by symptom remediation and habit reformation. Curious to see if this type of therapy should replace the current individual, once per week psychotherapy session, which focuses more on the psychodynamics behind the symptomatology, the Clinical Director authorized the development of a proposal to study the differential effectiveness of the two treatments. The initial plan for the study was to randomly select five of the homes that would switch to the newer treatment. All residents whose length of stay was less than three months at the time the study starts would be the focus of study, although due to the small atmosphere of the group homes, everyone would participate. Every subject in the study would be assessed every two months for one year, even after they returned to their community.

Applying Step One required the research associate to become more familiar with each form of treatment. After reading Lipsey (1993) and obtaining training manuals for the newer form of treatment, the researcher reviewed the literature for articles describing the effectiveness of each type of treatment. The use of abstracting services on CD-ROM drives at the University's library made these tasks easier to complete. After integrating the results of a meta-analysis of individual psychotherapy services with The Family Way's group home setting constraints, the researcher interviewed a random sample of group home staff members from three homes. The researcher asked about formal and informal program goals. Each participant also completed a brief survey of their expectations of what changes occur in residents during their stay and what is likely to happen for them once they return to the community.

The researcher shared these findings with the Clinical Director. Together they diagrammed the measurable inputs to treatment, the key treatment processes, and the most likely outcomes. The diagram in Figure 1 for the newer form of counseling indicated that the formation of one positive peer relationship during the group sessions was important. Provided this relationship grew outside of the sessions, then each group member's sense of well-being was likely to improve, due to the increase in positive experiences. Subsequently, as predicted by Howard et al.'s (1993) research, the symptoms of conduct disorder would decrease, followed by a decrease in behavioral problems. The minimum amount of time needed to accomplish a noticeable change in self-esteem was one month following the formation of this relationship.

The sequence of treatment steps recommended for brief individual psychotherapy for adolescents with conduct disorder was: (a) establish an accepting parent relationship, (b) clarify the feelings associated with behavioral problems as they occur, (c) identify a reward system for controlling a problem behavior and implement it, and (d) explore the buildup of negative feelings and how to handle them in advance of a violent incident. Usually several cycles of the first three steps occurred during the first six months of therapy, due to breakdowns in the therapeutic relationship. The last step seldom occurred before nine months of residential treatment were completed. Self-esteem was projected to fluctuate with each cycle and peak when a reward was received. Behavioral problems declined with each cycle. Symptoms of conduct disorder usually did not begin to recede until the fourth step was successfully implemented.

The researcher shared the diagrams with the management team, then with the quality of care committees at the three homes where staff participated in the prior survey. Based on the input received, the Clinical Director concluded that the effects of treatment should be tracked by measuring self-esteem, specific symptoms of conduct disorder, negative incidents, strength of peer relationships, overall satisfaction with life, and a parent or guardian's observations of adaptive functioning before and after the therapy.

The researcher then pondered possible unintended effects of each type of therapy, according to Step Two. One unintended effect of group counseling was mentioned in a journal article. The group often developed and pursued a group project to help the residential facility. When this occurred, reports of higher self-esteem were noted. Another unintended effect of group counseling was inferred from a systems analysis; the Clinical Director predicted the greater isolation of a few group members who did not form a closer relationship with a peer. They were likely to withdraw, perform fewer destructive acts while at the facility, then regress further upon release, behaving more aggressively upon returning to their community. One unintended effect of individual, brief psychotherapy was reported as greater social isolation from peers. Some patients tended to distance themselves from the group, as though disidentifying with the group's more destructive behavioral style. Another unintended effect of individual psychotherapy mentioned by several staff members was increasing depression. Since the depression effect was the only construct not already being considered, it was decided to add depression to the list.

Moving to Step Three, an assessment plan was created. The researcher obtained a copy of the article by Rosenblatt and Attkisson (1993). After drawing up a model similar to their three-dimensional model of domains, respondents, and contexts of measurement, the researcher and Clinical Director considered who needed to provide data and in which context other than the treatment facility. They made the following assignments, as depicted in Table 1.

Each row in Table 1 relates to one combination of a construct being measured by one type of respondent in either multiple contexts or a particular context within one domain. For example, depression is targeted as an indicator of clinical status. Reports from both the patient and the psychotherapist are of interest. Self-esteem is assigned to the Life Satisfaction domain, rather than the functional status domain; to the extent that the

TABLE 1. Outcome Assessment Plan for Remediation of Conduct Disorder

| Domain | Respondent | Context | Construct |
|---|---|---|---|
| Clinical | Patient | Individual | Depression |
| | Clinician | Individual | Depression Symptomatology |
| Functional | Patient | Multiple | Social Relations |
| | Clinician | Multiple | Social Relations |
| | Social Acq. | Multiple | Social Relations |
| | Family | Family | Adaptive Functioning |
| | | School | Adaptive Functioning |
| | | Community | Adaptive Functioning |
| Life Satisfaction | Patient | Multiple | Overall Satisfaction |
| | | Individual | Self-esteem |
| | Clinician | Individual | Self-esteem |
| Public Safety | Family | Multiple | Negative incidents |
| | Scientist | Multiple | Negative incidents |

researcher seeks a measure of satisfaction with one's self, this classification makes more sense, though the construct may be interpreted as an element of social competence (Heflinger, 1992). Negative incidents will be counted by research staff during the patient's stay at The Family Way group home. Negative incidents will also be estimated by a family member for two time periods, one prior to the patient's placement and the other following his return to the community. While it is possible to assess the same construct in different domains, such a situation did not arise in planning for this study.

Once the assessment plan took shape, the researcher began working on Step Four, searching for assessment instruments to add to the plan. Several of the sources of assessment instruments for children were consulted, as were recent articles in five journals. The Clinical Director also contributed several suggestions from her experience doing previous studies and by drawing upon a file of instruments compiled since obtaining her degree.

Referring to Table 1, two assessment instruments were needed for depression, one to be completed by the patient, the other by the treating clinician. The Interview Schedule for Children (Kovacs, 1983) and the Brief Psychiatric Rating Scale for Children (BPRS-C, Overall & Pfefferbaum, 1982) were readily identified as leading candidates. The BPRS-C was appealing because it also covers a wide range of symptoms. These two instruments were added to the assessment plan to cover all of the assessments of clinical status. Several longer inventories with scales for scoring depression, such as the Devereux Scales of Psychopathology (Naglieri et al., 1993), also were considered for covering clinical status, after reviewing suggestions by Hodges (1992) and by several authors who wrote chapters in Maruish (1994).

Two instruments stood out as the most attractive for obtaining a parent or guardian's report of adaptive functioning, the Child Behavior Checklist (CBCL, Achenbach, 1991) and Conners Parent Rating Scales (CPRS, Conners, 1989). No instrument was readily identified for reporting the strength of peer relationships, as viewed by patients or clinicians. Some suggestions provided by Nelson (1981) were noted for further consideration, such as self-monitoring and ad hoc self or other ratings. The research associate thought that forms could be developed and quickly piloted for wording choices, then included with the proposal for each type of respondent.

One measure of self-esteem recommended by Heflinger (1992) seemed satisfactory and was added to the list of measures, Harter's (1985) Self-perception Profile for Children. No formal assessment of overall satisfaction with life for adolescents was located. Based on some literature the researcher reviewed on adult measures, it was decided to use an adult measure with minor wording changes that would consist of two sentences requesting related overall judgments. Because each group home keeps a log of critical negative incidents, the log was listed as the measure for the scientist as respondent, i.e., the researcher. The directions for making entries in the log were revised to provide guidance for the parent or guardian, so they also could report on negative incidents before and after treatment.

Step Five, comparing alternative assessment instruments, was applied twice, once to decide among the instruments employed by a clinician to assess symptomatology and again to decide between the two assessments of adaptive functioning. Only the latter comparison is made here to illustrate the application of the ideal outcome assessment criteria.

It is recommended that copies of the instruments be obtained prior to making the comparisons, and applied to obtain some data. Whoever applies the instruments can be provided with the criteria, so they can contribute their impressions to the other information assembled. The researcher found two chapters in Maruish (1994) that covered most of the pertinent information about the two measures, relative to applying the 11 criteria. After applying each instrument himself to two patients, he formed the following impressions, which he discussed with the Clinical Director before choosing between instruments.

Both measures contained scales relating to conduct disorder and the response choices seemed relevant for assessing the patients at The Family Way. The researcher felt that the CBCL was more complicated to apply but the clear instructions tended to make the two assessments similar as to simple, teachable methods. Both instruments rely on adjectival anchors, making them roughly equivalent on the third criterion of types of referents supplied to respondents. Criterion Four, the use of multiple respondents, is better satisfied by the CBCL, although both instruments have versions for respondents other than parent or guardian. With no plans for utilizing two or more reports of adaptive functioning, this criterion was dropped from consideration. Both the researcher and the Clinical Director concluded that the CBCL's coverage of social problems might help identify a key treatment process diagrammed in Step One. Thus, this instrument seemed to have an edge on Criterion Five.

The psychometric strength of both instruments was high and extensively documented. Test-retest reliability and internal consistency appeared higher across scales for the CBCL. Less information was available about the validity of the CPRS for parents, although several studies have shown its ability to distinguish among clinical groups and clinical from control groups. The content validity of the CBCL seemed good, according to the manual. Also, more studies of the CBCL's sensitivity to treatment-related change have been performed. Both instruments are vulnerable to biasing influences on rater behavior. The CPRS is known to experience some inflation of scores with repeated assessments. Care should be taken to compare scores on both instruments with other data about the same patient to check for potential biasing effects. Given the sizable correlations between corresponding scales on these two instruments, there may not be any critical differences in psychometric strength between the two. However, after weighing the evidence available, it seemed the CBCL tended to perform better.

The costs of applying either instrument were broken down into acquisition cost, administration, data storage, scoring, and utilization of results. It was decided that a paper and pencil form would be mailed to the parent or guardian and a telephone interview conducted to help that person complete the form. While the ease of scoring the CPRS by hand offered savings over the CBCL in data storage and scoring, the availability of computerized scoring programs for the CBCL was considered a lower-cost way to quickly utilize the results. The purchase fee for the CBCL seemed like a higher cost except that the cost of staff time spent duplicating the CPRS was expected to offset that disadvantage. Across all costs, it appeared that the CPRS held a slight advantage.

Due to the similarities in scales and score profiles across instruments, the conclusion was reached that there would be minimal differences between instruments on the last four criteria–understanding by nonprofessional audiences, ease of providing feedback, usefulness in clinical services, and compatibility with clinical theories and practices. To choose between instruments, the first seven criteria were weighted equally. The CBCL was selected for inclusion in the study design because it was preferred on two criteria to one for the CPRS. A subsequent analysis of the results was performed for an unequal weighting scheme, in which costs and psychometric strength were highly weighted. Due to the offsetting advantages of lower cost for the CPRS and higher psychometric strength for the CBCL, the choice of the CBCL was not reversed.

Under the circumstances described in connection with this hypothetical example, there was neither the time nor resources to perform a more formal analysis of the differences in attractiveness between assessment instruments. Under less constrained circumstances, procedures such as the one employed by Green and Gracely (1987) for collecting and analyzing data about each criterion should be considered. When the circumstances are even more constrained, a more cavalier approach to making comparisons is preferable to simply choosing an instrument with a reputation. The development of this example describes the value of applying the selection criteria, as well as attending to all five steps in the process. Even though one's preferences are global judgments, the more thoroughly the available information is scrutinized, the more likely that all relevant issues will be surfaced and addressed before a choice is made.

Since the selection of appropriate outcome measures is critical to obtaining informative research data (Pfeiffer, 1989), it is recommended that researchers always try to apply the above five steps utilizing the 11 ideal outcome measure criteria. Typically, the time available for applying the five steps is inadequate. Also, there are other important decisions to be made when planning for and conducting research on the effectiveness of residential treatments that consume time (Attkisson et al., 1978; Durkin & Durkin, 1975; Pfeiffer, 1989). Because the amount of time available is always an issue, we expect that researchers will emphasize one or two of the decisions being made during the design and conduct of each study of residential treatments. In designing subsequent studies, the same researcher will likely emphasize different decisions. One solution to the problem of a lack of time is to emphasize gathering more information relating to those research study decisions for which the researcher lacks knowledge. Whenever the focus on outcomes shifts, though, consider familiarizing oneself with the most appropriate outcome measures.

## REFERENCES

Achenbach, T. M. (1991). *Manual for the Child Behavior Checklist/4-18 and 1991 profile.* Burlington, VT: University of Vermont, Department of Psychiatry.

Ackoff, R. (1975). *Redesigning the future.* New York: John Wiley and Sons.

Attkisson, C. C., Hargreaves, W. A., Horowitz, M. J., & Sorensen, J. E. (Eds.) (1978). *Evaluation of human service programs.* New York: Academic Press.

Conners, C. K. (1989). *Manual for Conners Rating Scales.* N. Tonawanda, NY: Multi-Health Systems.

Durkin, R. P., & Durkin, A. B. (1975). Evaluating residential treatment programs for disturbed children. In M. Guttentag & E. L. Struening (Eds.), *Handbook of evaluation research* (Vol. 2). Beverly Hills: Sage Publications.

Green, R. S., & Gracely, E. J. (1987). Selecting a rating scale for evaluating services to the chronically mentally ill. *Community Mental Health Journal, 23,* 91-102.

Hammill, D. D., Brown, L., & Bryant, B. R. (1992). *A consumer's guide to tests in print* (2nd ed.). Austin, TX: Proed.

Harter, S. (1985). *Manual for the Self-perception Profile for Children.* Denver, CO: Department of Psychology, University of Denver.

Heflinger, C. A. (1992). Client-level outcomes of mental health services for children and adolescents. In L. Bickman & D. J. Rog (Eds.), *Evaluating mental health services for children: No. 54. New directions for program evaluation* (pp. 31-46). San Francisco: Jossey-Bass Publishers.

Hodges, K. (1992). Diagnosis and symptomatology. In L. Bickman & D. J. Rog (Eds.), *Evaluating mental health services for children: No. 54. New directions for program evaluation* (pp. 47-56). San Francisco: Jossey-Bass Publishers.

House, E. R. (1980). *Evaluating with validity.* Beverly Hills: Sage Publications.

Howard, K. I., Lueger, R. J., Maling, M. S., & Zoran, M. (1993). A phase model of psychotherapy outcome: Causal mediation of change. *Journal of Consulting and Clinical Psychology, 61,* 678-685.

Johnson, O. G. (Ed.). (1976). *Tests and measurements in child development: Handbook II* (2 Vols.). San Francisco: Jossey-Bass.

Johnson, O. G., Bommarito, J. W. (Eds.). (1971). *Tests and measurements in child development: A handbook.* San Francisco: Jossey-Bass.

Kovacs, M. (1983). *The Interview Schedule for Children (ISC): ISC interrater and parent-child agreement.* Pittsburgh, PA: Department of Psychiatry, University of Pittsburgh School of Medicine.

Krug, S. E. (1987). *Psychware sourcebook: 1987-1988* (2nd ed.). Champaign, IL: Metritech Inc.

Lawrence, J. E. S., & Cook, T. J. (1982). Designing useful evaluations: The stakeholder survey. *Evaluation and Program Planning, 5,* 327-336.

Lipsey, M. W. (1993). Theory as method: Small theories of treatments. In L. B. Sechrest & A. G. Scott (Eds.), *Understanding causes and generalizing about them. No. 57. New directions for program evaluation* (pp. 5-38). San Francisco: Jossey Bass Publishers.

Maruish, M. E. (Ed.). (1994). *The use of psychological testing for treatment planning and outcome assessment.* Hillsdale, NJ: Lawrence Erlbaum Associates, Publishers.

National Institute of Mental Health (1983). *Series AN No. 1. The assessment of psychopathology and behavioral problems in children: A review of scales suitable for epidemiological and clinical research, 1967-1979* (DHHS Publication No. ADM 83-1037). Washington, DC: U.S. Government Printing Office.

National Institute of Mental Health (1984). *Series AN No. 3. The assessment of adaptive functioning in children: A review of existing measures suitable for epidemiological and clinical research* (DHHS Publication No. ADM 84-1343). Washington, DC: U.S. Government Printing Office.

Nelson, R. O. (1981). Realistic dependent measures for clinical use. *Journal of Consulting and Clinical Psychology, 49,* 168-182.

Newman, F. L. & Ciarlo, J. A. (1994). Criteria for selecting psychological instruments for treatment outcome assessment. In M. E. Maruish (Ed.), *The use of psychological testing for treatment planning and outcome assessment* (pp. 98-110). Hillsdale, NJ: Lawrence Erlbaum Associates, Publishers.

Newman, F. L., Fitt, D., & Heverly, M. A. (1987). Influences of patient, service program and clinician characteristics on judgments of functioning and treatment recommendations. *Evaluation and Program Planning, 10,* 260-267.

Newman, F. L., Kopta, S. M., McGovern, M. P., Howard, K. I., & McNeilly, C. (1988). Evaluating the conceptualizations and treatment plans of interns and supervisors during a psychology internship. *Journal of Consulting and Clinical Psychology, 56,* 659-665.

Overall, J. E., & Pfefferbaum, B. (1982). The Brief Psychiatric Rating Scale for Children. *Psychopharmacology Bulletin, 18,* 10-16.

Rosenblatt, A., & Attkisson, C. C. (1993). Assessing outcomes for sufferers of severe mental disorders: A conceptual framework and review. *Evaluation and Program Planning, 16,* 347-364.

Pfeiffer, S. I. (1989). Follow-up of children and adolescents treated in psychiatric facilities: A methodology review. *The Psychiatric Hospital, 20,* 15-20.

Pfeiffer, S. I., Soldivera, S., & Norton, J. (1992). *A consumer's guide to mental health treatment outcome measures.* Devon, PA: The Devereux Foundation.

Sherrill, S. (1984). Identifying and measuring unintended outcomes. *Evaluation and Program Planning, 7,* 27-34.

Stewart, B. J., & Archbold, P. G. (1992). Nursing intervention studies require outcome measures that are sensitive to change: Part One. *Research in Nursing & Health, 15,* 477-481.

Stewart, B. J., & Archbold, P. G. (1993). Nursing intervention studies require outcome measures that are sensitive to change: Part Two. *Research in Nursing & Health, 16,* 77-81.

Suchman, E. A. (1967). *Evaluative research.* New York: Russell Sage Foundation.

Sweetland, R. C., & Keyser, D. J. (Eds.). (1991). *Tests* (3rd ed.). Kansas City, KS: Test Corporation of America.

Webb, E. J., Campbell, D. T., Schwartz, R. D., & Sechrest, L. (1966). *Unobtrusive measures: Nonreactive research in the social sciences.* Chicago: Rand McNally.

# A Comparison of Commonly Used Treatment Measures

## D. Patrick Zimmerman, Psyd

**SUMMARY.** This commentary briefly surveys some of the practical and methodological difficulties related to residential treatment outcome research, both in terms of earlier criticisms of outcome research and of more recent commentaries noting the increased importance of funding issues and fiscal accountability. The paper concludes with a descriptive and comparative survey listing of selected possible outcome assessment instruments, including: (1) clinical interview schedules, (2) objective rating scales (including global functioning, behavioral, and specialized focus scales), (3) objective personality inventories, and (4) projective tests. *[Article copies available from The Haworth Document Delivery Service: 1-800-342-9678. E-mail address: getinfo@haworth.com]*

### INTRODUCTION

Other papers in this collection of essays on the general theme of outcome assessment for residential treatment discuss historical perspectives

D. Patrick Zimmerman is Coordinator of Research and Lecturer, The Department of Psychiatry, at the Sonia Shankman Orthogenic School at the University of Chicago. He teaches psychodiagnostic assessment courses in the Committee on Human Development, the University of Chicago, and at the Illinois School for Professional Psychology, where he is a member of the Associate Core Faculty. Dr. Zimmerman is a Candidate at the Chicago Center for Psychoanalysis.

[Haworth co-indexing entry note]: "A Comparison of Commonly Used Treatment Measures." Zimmerman, D. Patrick. Co-published simultaneously in *Residential Treatment for Children & Youth* (The Haworth Press, Inc.) Vol. 13, No. 4, 1996, pp. 49-69; and: *Outcome Assessment in Residential Treatment* (ed: Steven I. Pfeiffer) The Haworth Press, Inc., 1996, pp. 49-69. Single or multiple copies of this article are available from The Haworth Document Delivery Service [1-800-342-9678, 9:00 a.m. - 5:00 p.m. (EST). E-mail address: getinfo@haworth.com].

on outcome assessment, the necessity and goals of such evaluation, the process of choosing particular instruments, and the clinical implications of residential outcome assessment. Nevertheless, a brief reconsideration of some of those issues is of value for the present discussion of residential treatment outcome evaluation, which focuses upon a descriptive and comparative listing of selected, but sometimes frequently utilized, assessment instruments. It should be noted that, partly due to space limitations, this discussion is limited to personality and behavioral assessment instruments; it does not review intelligence tests such as the Stanford-Binet, WISC-III, WAIS-R, and the Kaufman-ABC, although intelligence estimates can certainly play an important part in descriptions of residential treatment outcome.

## RECENT DISCUSSIONS OF RESIDENTIAL TREATMENT OUTCOME ASSESSMENT

For many years a number of writers decried the paucity of sophisticated research on the long-term effects of inpatient and residential treatment for the psychiatrically disturbed adolescent (Garber, 1972; Gossett, Lewis, & Barnhart, 1983; Hartmann, Glasser, Greenblatt, Soloman, & Levinson, 1968; Klinge, Piggot, Knitter, & O'Donnell, 1986). Further, the available outcome research was said to be difficult to compare, due to a number of methodological differences. Garber (1972) noted that earlier studies utilized a variety of treatment methods, were often unclear about criteria for measuring improvement, had different foci (e.g., diagnosis, sample description, disposition, or current level of functioning), and frequently treated "the therapeutic modalities employed during the hospital stay . . . as an afterthought." Wilson and Lyman (1983) surveyed evaluation research in residential treatment in terms of outcome measures, treatment effects, research design, subject characteristics, and systems considerations. They proposed that the attempt to arrive at a conclusive statement about the effectiveness of residential treatment was analogous to making a similar prediction about psychotherapy. They concluded from their review that "the investigation of residential treatment has not been such that there is anything approaching a science or a clear model of what works" (Wilson & Lyman, 1983, p. 1085).

More recent commentaries on the status of residential treatment followup evaluation have discussed issues such as the goals of outcome assessment, problems facing the implementation of evaluation research programs, ways in which such problems might be surmounted, and the relative importance of statistically-oriented evaluation research as compared to more qualitative, hypothesis-generating studies. While most authors see the evaluation of treatment effectiveness as the major manifest goal for outcome assessment, such effectiveness is being viewed more frequently within what is often seen as the more crucial underlying contexts of "cost effectiveness," the attainment and maintenance of funding for mental health services, and accountability to funding agents, "market forces," and payers' evaluations of the quality of care being provided (Curry, 1995; Prentice-Dunn & Lyman, 1989; Vermillion & Pfeiffer, 1993). This increased stress upon financial issues appears to have been accompanied by some de-emphasis on the type of residential treatment research which is more directly related to the human domain of developmental psychopathology, conducted either for its own sake as an exploratory contribution to clinical understanding or carried out as an important component of residential outcome research.

In addition to the variety of problems facing residential treatment research already described, more recently published discussions have noted a number of other practical and methodological obstacles. For example, one survey of 273 residential treatment clinicians revealed that, despite the respondents' overwhelmingly favorable attitudes about the importance of research, the clinicians reported what seemed to be relatively formidable practical obstacles to actually conducting research in their work settings (Pfeiffer, S., Burd, S., & Wright, A., 1992). These barriers included such basic, practical issues as a lack of sufficient time, lack of institutional funding for research, and institutional reluctance to designate research as a formal part of clinicians' work responsibilities.

An important and long-standing methodological issue is the continuing debate between those who view the statistical significance of a hypothetico-deductive approach as a superordinate goal in outcome research (with its preoccupations with large samples, randomized designs, statistical hypotheses, and strivings to "scientifically prove" treatment effectiveness), as opposed to those who question the clinical value of such efforts and who instead view inductive and even qualitative residential treatment research approaches as having made the *major* contributions to our understanding of youth in residential care (Mordock, in press). Notable studies representing the latter view, based upon the multi-dimensional qualitative case study approach to follow-up assessment, include a major Chestnut Lodge study of schizophrenia, treatment process, and outcome (McGlashan & Keats, 1989), and the Menninger Clinic's follow-up study of 48 patients in psychoanalysis and psychotherapy (Wallerstein, 1986).

Other methodological difficulties recently noted by various authors have included the continuing problem of specifying programmatic components of residential care as clearly defined and measurable treatment interventions, failures to study the milieu in a rigorous manner, and the paucity of residential outcome research presenting clear measurement of actual treatment implementation (Curry, 1995; Mordock, in press; Prentice-Dunn & Lyman, 1989). Further, some authors have described problems such as inadequate demographic descriptions of the specific populations in residential treatment settings and the difficulty in selecting valid and reliable formal assessment instruments, related both to the demographic indicants of a particular residential setting's population and to formal outcome measures of treatment effectiveness (Prentice-Dunn & Lyman, 1989). This issue of the difficulty in choosing reliable and valid assessment instruments is, of course, of special importance for this paper.

Fortunately, at this point there are a number of comprehensive, standard reference texts of particular value in evaluating the psychometric qualities and usefulness of specific assessment instruments. These resource texts include: *Tests in Print III* (Mitchell, 1983); *The Mental Measurements Yearbook* (Conoley & Kramer, 1989); *Tests: A Comprehensive Reference for Assessment in Psychology, Education and Business* (Sweetland & Keyser, 1991); *Test Critiques* (Keyser & Sweetland, 1985); and *Measures of Personality and Social Psychological Attitudes* (Robinson, Shaver & Wrightsman, 1991).

Other quite useful descriptive guides to frequently used assessment instruments include: *A Consumer's Guide to Tests in Print, 2nd Ed.* (Hammill, Brown, & Bryant, 1992), *A Consumer's Guide to Mental Health Treatment Outcome Measures* (Pfeiffer, Soldivera, & Norton, 1992), and *Measures for Clinical Practice, Vols. I and II, 2nd Ed.* (Fischer & Corcoran, 1994). It should be noted that in the face of the difficulty in selecting useful outcome assessment tools, many writers have strongly emphasized the importance of developing an outcome evaluation program which is multi-dimensional and multi-perspective, utilizing a *variety* of assessment tools (Prentice-Dunn & Lyman, 1989; Vermillion & Pfeiffer, 1993; Whittaker, Overstreet, Grasso, Tripodi, & Boylan, 1988).

## *A SELECTIVE DESCRIPTIVE LISTING*
## *OF OUTCOME ASSESSMENT MEASURES*

While it is far beyond the scope of this paper to present a comprehensive and detailed picture of the range of available evaluation tools available to the clinician, it is possible to provide a picture of various categories of available instruments through a relatively brief comparison and description of a few of the more well known psychological instruments. The selected test descriptions are written for a broad intended readership, hopefully balancing the needs of both clinicians interested in outcome research with those of other residential treatment direct-care workers who might be interested in achieving a basic familiarity with psychological tests.

Many of the tests described here are among the most frequently used instruments in the assessment of youth, as suggested by the report of a survey of 165 American Psychological Association clinicians regarding personality assessment measures used with adolescents (Archer, Maruish, Imhof, & Piotrowski, 1991). Table 1 shows the top 20 psychological assessment instruments mentioned in the survey, as well as each test's weighted score rank based upon the frequency of use. It is of interest to note that only one objective personality test, the MMPI, was among the top ten most frequently used instruments in adolescent assessment batteries, while seven of the top ten tests were projective personality instruments.

The following survey of possible outcome assessment instruments includes descriptions of selected (1) clinical interview schedules, (2) objective rating scales (including global functioning, behavioral, and special-

TABLE 1. Frequency of Use of Psychodiagnostic Instruments with Adolescents

| Weighted Score Rank | Instrument |
| --- | --- |
| 1 | WISC-R/WAIS-R |
| 2 | Rorschach |
| 3 | Bender-Gestalt |
| 4 | Thematic Apperception Test |
| 5 | Sentence Completion |
| 6 | MMPI |
| 7 | Human Figure Drawing |
| 8 | House-Tree-Person |
| 9 | Wide Range Achievement Test |
| 10 | Kinetic Family Drawing |
| 11 | Beck Depression Inventory |
| 12 | Millon Adol. Personality Inventory |
| 13 | MacAndrew Alcoholism Scale |
| 14 | Child Behavior Checklist |
| 15 | Woodcock Johnson |
| 16 | Peabody Picture Vocabulary Test |
| 17 | Conners Behavior Rating Scale |
| 18 | Beery VMI |
| 19 | Reynolds Adol. Depression Scale |
| 20 | Children's Depression Inventory |

ized focus scales), (3) objective personality inventories, and (4) projective tests. The listing briefly describes each instrument's general structure, intended subject group, stated purpose or goal, psychometrics, and, when applicable, special considerations related to use of the instrument. Psychometric evaluations are presented only in a general manner, and readers are urged to consult some of the previously mentioned guides to tests in print for greater psychometric detail.

## I. Structured Interviews

Structured (and semi-structured) clinical interview schedules are administered orally by the clinician and require the cooperative responses of the child or adolescent, and in some cases the parent. The goal of this type of instrument is usually to gain an estimate of the youth's current coping skills, symptomatology, and diagnosis. Factors influencing the usefulness of this assessment tool include: the level and quality of the clinician's interview experience, guardedness as a factor in the youth's self-report responses, parental attitudes toward the youth reflected in the parent responses, and resistance to the lengthy and time-consuming interview format. Further, the general psychometric qualities of all the instruments described below (in terms of both reliability and validity) is doubtful.

Finally, to the extent that this type of assessment instrument focuses on specifying a particular diagnosis, it should be taken into account that however specific a diagnosis might be, the term can never denote a precise constellation of symptoms which occurs independent of other symptoms. Thus, use of an interview schedule alone in outcome assessment cannot realistically capture the complexities of psychological functioning, nor can it adequately provide more than an incomplete picture of personality change related to treatment, since no single measure of dysfunction can routinely capture the psychological complexity of the youth being assessed.

1. *Child Assessment Schedule (CAS).* The Child Assessment Schedule (Hodges, Kline, Fitch, McKnew, & Cytryn, 1981) is clinician administered to the child or parent. It is a lengthy interview schedule, with 320 total items requiring an administration time of between 45 to 90 minutes. It is appropriate for use with youth between the ages of 7 and 14 years of age and aims to assess the level of coping skills, onset and duration of symptomatology, and diagnosis. The length of this schedule may make administration difficult with either easily distractible, hyperactive, or seriously disturbed youth.

2. *Diagnostic Interview for Children and Adolescents (DICA)*. The Diagnostic Interview for Children and Adolescents (Herjanic & Campbell, 1977) is a frequently reported instrument in the research literature which focuses upon the nature of and treatment outcomes of particular psychological disorders. It is clinician administered to the youth/ parent, and is appropriate for use with youth from 6 to 17 years of age. The schedule consists of 267-311 yes/no questions and requires 1 1/2 hours to administer. The major purpose of this instrument is the assessment of psychiatric symptomatology, especially related to specific diagnostic categories. As with the other interview schedules described here, the length of the interview may make administration difficult with some youth in distress.

3. *Psychiatric Status Schedule (PSS)*. The Psychiatric Status Schedule (Spitzer, Endicott, Fleiss, & Cohen, 1970) is administered by the clinician to the child and is composed of 321 items requiring 30-50 minutes to administer. Its major focus is upon role functioning and (mostly) affective symptomatology. The extensive pool of 321 items suggests that administration to some children may present significant difficulties, similar to those mentioned in descriptions of the previous two interview schedules.

## II. Rating Scales

The different types of rating scales offer both unique advantages in outcome assessment, as well as a variety of obstacles. For example, the global functioning scales are extremely time-efficient, requiring the clinician simply to choose either a single rating from a continuum of numbers related to level of functioning, or to make Likert format choices on more than one scale of functioning. On the other hand, rating decisions may be highly influenced by clinician subjectivity and the ratings yield only gross estimates of functioning, hopelessly unable to capture the complexity of psychological functioning. As a result, the psychometric quality of global assessment measures has generally been described as unacceptable.

Other significant assessment problems are presented by behavioral and specialized rating scales. While the face objectivity of their formats may mislead clinicians into unquestioned acceptance of their psychometric soundness, the results of some recent personality research projects have raised the possibility of serious limitations to the soundness of the psychological conclusions suggested by such rating scales.

For example, in a study of the psychological functioning of sexually abused children, Leifer, Shapiro, Martone, and Kassem (1991) pointed out that a major limitation of many studies of the short-term psychological effects of child sexual abuse has been a reliance on either child self-report measures or on parental reports of the child's behavioral difficulties. Such measures appear to be highly subject to distortion in this population, and often provide discrepant results. In a number of studies utilizing self-report assessment measures, sexually abused children were frequently not significantly distinguished from normative groups with regard to indicators of depression, anxiety, or self-esteem (Belter, Lipovsky, & Finch, 1989; McLeer, Deblinger, Atkins, Foa, & Ralphe, 1988; Shapiro, Leifer, Martone, & Kassem, 1990; Tong, Oates, & McDowell, 1987). Leifer et al. (1991, p. 15) pointed out that one explanation for these seemingly unlikely results may be that sexually abused children may be highly guarded and either unwilling or unable to disclose their painful internal states in the self-report assessment situation, an explanation that might also hold true for a broad range of emotionally distressed youth.

The low correspondence between parent and child ratings is also well reported in the literature. Parental reports may reflect factors other than objective measures of the child's functioning, such as the parent's own level of distress (Friedrich & Reams, 1987; Kazdin, French, & Unis, 1983; Moretti, Fine, Haley, and Marriage, 1985) or the degree of emotional support they characteristically are able or willing to provide for the child (Everson, Hunter, Runyon, Edelsohn, & Coulter, 1989). All these findings strongly suggest the need to utilize additional psychological assessment measures which are capable both of bypassing children's reluctance to reveal painful internal states and of focusing on non-behavioral processes effected by a child's psychological state.

*A. Global Functioning Scales*

1. *Global Assessment Scale (GAS).* The Global Assessment Scale (Endicott, Spitzer, Fleiss, & Cohen, 1976) is a single-point rating scale based upon a continuum of 1 to 100, where higher scores suggest better levels of social and psychological functioning. The rating is quick and based upon clinician judgment. It provides a gross estimate of functioning in areas such as severity of observable symptomatology, inferences of subjective distress, behavioral disturbances, and reality testing. As mentioned earlier, this scale provides only a general quantitative estimate of functioning, is vulnerable to clinician subjectivity, and has questionable psychometric value.

2. *Children's Global Assessment Scale (CGAS).* The Children's Global Assessment Scale (Shaffer, Gould, Brasie, Ambrosini, Fisher, Bird, & Aluwahilia, 1983) is an adaptation for children of the GAS and is intended for use in assessing the functioning of children 4-16 years

of age. It is similar in format and purpose to the GAS described above and, therefore, shares the difficulties of evaluator subjectivity, lack of diagnostic or syndrome specificity, and lack of verified psychometric rigor.

3. *Timberlawn Child Functioning Scale (TCFS)*. The Timberlawn Child Functioning Scale (Dimperio, Blotcky, Gossett, & Doyle, 1986) has a Likert-type format for clinician response on 14 scales related to cognitive, affective, and social functioning. It is intended for use with both children and adolescents, and yields a general estimate of a child's adaptive level over the previous year. As with the GAS and CGAS, reliance on the assessment conclusions based upon administration of the TCFS should be tempered by an awareness of the possible influence of rater subjectivity, lack of syndrome specificity, and questionable psychometric integrity.

*B. Behavior Rating Scales*

1. *Child Behavior Checklist (CBCL)*. The Child Behavior Checklist (Achenbach, 1991a, 1991b) is one of the more frequently cited assessment instruments in follow-up research reports. The CBCL is a 118 item behavioral scale for children and adolescents from 4-18 years of age, and it focuses on behaviors related to social and emotional problems. The CBCL is completed either by youth self-report or by the parent, can be completed in only 15-17 minutes, and has generally good psychometric properties. Nevertheless, potential drawbacks to the use of this instrument in outcome assessment include: a focus which is mainly upon a range of manifest, observable behaviors, rather than upon issues of intrapsychic functioning; conclusions may be influenced by self-report guardedness or parental biases, and the required 5th grade reading level can be an obstacle in administration to subjects with language and/or reading difficulties.

2. *Conners' Parent Rating Scale (CPRS)*. The Conners' Parent Rating Scale (Conners, 1989) is a 93 item test, arranged on a 4 point scale to measure severity of each behavior. Completed by parents (a teacher's form is also available), it is applicable for children and adolescents from 3 to 17 years of age. The CPRS requires a 30 minute administration time, but shorter versions are available for both the parent and teacher forms. However, reviews of psychometric quality for this scale are variable, ranging from unacceptable to adequate/acceptable. In addition, as with the CBCL, the focus of this instrument is almost solely upon externalized behaviors, to the neglect of the internal realm of symptoms and disorders.

3. *Devereux Scales of Mental Disorders (DSMD).* The Devereux Scales of Mental Disorders (Naglieri, LeBuffe, & Pfeiffer, 1994) is a 110 item checklist, with a 5-point scale for each item. It is available in two versions (child/adolescent) and is useful with children 5-12 years old and with adolescents 13-18 years old. The DSMD can be completed by a parent, teacher, or other adult familiar with the youth's behavior in a home-like or educational setting. Administration time is only 15 minutes, and the instrument claims both to evaluate certain types of psychopathology, behavioral problems and to measure behavioral changes. The DSMD is composed of items based on current DSM-IV definitions, and both reliability and validity properties for this instrument are said to range from adequate to good.

4. *Eyberg Child Behavior Inventory (ECBI).* The Eyberg Child Behavior Inventory (Eyberg, 1992) is a 36 item behavioral rating scale to be used with youth from 2 to 16 years of age. It assesses behavioral problems and rates the intensity of those behaviors. The focus of this scale is limited to conduct problems and behavioral enactments; in addition, the psychometric qualities of this instrument are questionable.

5. *Jesness Behavior Checklist (JBC).* The Jesness Behavior Checklist (Jesness, 1984) is an 80 item, 5 point scale, yielding an observer's or self-rated evaluation of problem behaviors in youth from 13 to 21 years of age. As with the ECBI, its purpose is very limited in scope, i.e., the screening and assessment of delinquent behaviors. In addition, while the instrument appears to be predictive of future arrests for delinquent behavior, other measures of psychometric standing for this instrument are less than adequate.

6. *Louisville Behavioral Checklist (LBCL).* The Louisville Behavioral Checklist (Miller, 1984) is a wide-ranging behavioral checklist, with four forms for use with children and adolescents from ages 4-17. Completed by a parent within a 20-30 minute administration period, the main purpose of the test is to serve as a screening instrument for problem behaviors. Reliability levels for this test are variable, and validity is questionable. The adolescent version has three notable problems: inadequate validity research, a lack of norms, and a required 10th grade reading level. The latter demand may clearly put certain groups of parents at a distinct disadvantage in their efforts to accurately respond to this version of the LBCL.

## C. Specialized Rating Scales

1. *Children's Depression Inventory (CDI).* The Children's Depression Inventory (Kovacs, 1992) is, as with the CBCL, one of the more frequently cited instruments in research focusing on children's psychological functioning and outcome assessment. The CDI is a self-report, 27 item forced-choice inventory for 7 to 17 year old youth and takes 15 minutes or less to administer. The inventory is aimed toward the specific assessment of depression, as reflected in the dimensions of affective behavior, ideation, interpersonal relations, and feelings of guilt and irritability. Some psychometric properties of the CDI are questionable, and assessment reached by this test is vulnerable to influence by subject factors such as guardedness in the self-report responses.

2. *Coopersmith Self-Esteem Inventories (SEI).* The Coopersmith Self-Esteem Inventories (Coopersmith, 1987) are self-report inventories published in two forms, the School form (58 items, 8-15 years of age) and the Adult form (25 items, 16 years and older). The instruments yield measures of self-attitude with regard to social, academic, and interpersonal experiences. Advantages include a brief administration time (10 minutes) and, for the School form, generally good psychometric properties. Serious caution should be exercised in the use of the Adult form for outcome assessment with adolescents 16 years and older for two significant reasons: (1) the psychometric soundness of this version is unknown, since there is no reliability or validity data available for the Adult form and (2) the norms for the Adult form are based on a small and generally unrepresentative sample of 226 college students.

3. *Piers-Harris Children's Self-Concept Scale (Piers-Harris).* The Piers-Harris (Piers, 1984) is an 80 "yes/no" item self-report inventory of self-concept attitudes related to such functional categories as behavior, perceived intellect and school performance, physical attributes, and perceived quality of peer relations. It is intended for use with youth from 8-18 years of age, and requires a relatively brief administration time (15-20 minutes). The general psychometric quality of the Piers-Harris is suspect; in particular, outcome assessment researchers should use this instrument with caution, since the normative sample is outdated, not representative, and inadequately described.

4. *Tennessee Self-Concept Scale (TSCS).* The Tennessee Self-Concept Scale (Roid & Fitts, 1988) is a 100 item self-report scale, with a relatively brief administration time of 10-20 minutes. It is intended for

use with subjects 12 years of age and older and measures a number of self-concept variables, including: identity, behavior, self-satisfaction, family relationships, and social relations. Although the reported general psychometric qualities of the TSCS range from good to excellent, researchers evaluating a residential treatment population should note the fact that college level students are over-represented in the normative sample of this instrument.

### III. Objective Personality Inventories

Empirically-based objective or structured personality tests were originally developed partially in response to the criticism that projective assessment instruments were too subjective and lacked psychometric soundness. It is true that objective personality instruments, especially tests such as the Minnesota Multiphasic Personality Inventory, the Millon Clinical Multiaxial Inventory, and the Millon Adolescent Personality Inventory, have represented the standard for statistical soundness in testing. While usually psychometrically sound, objective personality instruments tend to yield a diagnosis-oriented assessment, with profile personality interpretations being somewhat general and inferential (i.e., "this person's personality functioning is probably similar to others who present a similar or identical scale profile"), rather than being specifically derived from and unique to the internal psychodynamics of the particular individual being assessed.

1. *Jesness Inventory.* The Jesness Inventory (Jesness, 1988) is a 155 true/false item self-report personality inventory for use with 8-19 year-old youth, with a particular focus on issues of delinquency. While it has been said to be discriminant between nondelinquent and delinquent subjects and predictive of future criminal activity, some aspects of this inventory's reliability and validity are questionable.

2. *Millon Adolescent Personality Inventory (MAPI) and the Millon Adolescent Clinical Inventory (MACI).* The Millon Adolescent Personality Inventory (Millon, Green, & Meagher, 1982), because of its construction and sensitivity qualities, has been viewed by some professionals and researchers as the adolescent assessment instrument of choice. It is a 150 true-false item self-report instrument that identifies eight personality styles, eight concerns frequently expressed by adolescents, and four scales highlighting behaviors of particular interest to clinicians and school personnel. The recently developed Millon Adolescent Clinical Inventory is more clinically oriented than the MAPI and evaluates maladaptive levels of twelve personal-

ity styles, including the eight previously included in the MAPI. The MACI also provides information on adolescent expressed concerns and nine clinical indices of maladjusted behaviors. The MAPI has adequate general psychometric properties, and similar levels are claimed for the MACI. A limitation of both of these structured personality tests is that there are a multitude of individual differences found between subjects with seemingly similar profiles. Researchers who recognize this limitation will understand that the results of statistically valuable objective instruments such as the MAPI and MACI are more valuable in outcome assessment when *integrated* into a multi-dimensional battery of assessment instruments.

3. *The Minnesota Multiphasic Personality Inventory-Adolescent (MMPI-A).* The original self-report MMPI has been described as the most frequently referenced and psychometrically sound personality assessment instrument. The MMPI-A (Butcher, Williams, Graham, Archer, Tellegen, Ben-Porath, & Kaemmer, 1992) is a revision of the original MMPI and is particularly designed for use with youth between the ages of 12 and 18. However, caution should be used in the administration of the MMPI-A to 12 and 13-year-old subjects, who tend to produce substantially different norms than the central 14 through 18-year-old group of adolescents. In addition the group of 12 and 13-year-old youth will inevitably contain many subjects unable to successfully read and understand the MMPI-A item pool.

The MMPI-A is a 478-item true/false measure. The original MMPI basic clinical scales and self-report format have been retained in the MMPI-A. These basic scales tend to emphasize diagnostic syndromes and symptomatology. In addition, the MMPI-A represents an attempt to improve the original MMPI with regard to adolescent assessment, and revisions include: a reduction in the total number of items, revision of a number of items to improve wording, and the development of several new scales said to be particularly associated with adolescent development and psychopathology. Ongoing validity and reliability research on the MMPI-A suggests variable reliability (low to moderate, depending upon the particular clinical scale being considered), although factor analytic findings for the MMPI-A are reasonably consistent with prior factor analytic findings reported for adolescent populations on the original MMPI. Parents of adolescents used in the MMPI-A normative sample clearly over-represent higher educational levels in comparison with the general U.S. population. Continued psychometric research on the MMPI-A will be useful.

Limitations on use of the MMPI-A with some distractible or disturbed adolescents are posed by the length of this self-report test (nearly 500 items) and the required seventh-grade reading level. In addition, the MMPI-A shares certain interpretive difficulties with the MAPI, specifically that there are in fact a multitude of psychological and behavioral differences between subjects who present seemingly similar test profiles. As with the MAPI, researchers who recognize this limitation of the instrument will realize that the clinical picture provided by the MMPI-A is much more valuable in outcome assessment when *integrated* into a battery of assessment instruments.

## IV. Projective Personality Instruments

Over the years, researchers have tended to avoid the use of projective personality tests in outcome assessment due to major problems associated with variations in administration procedures, clinician subjectivity regarding interpretation, and a lack of psychometric integrity. Nevertheless, projective instruments characteristically appear to have the dual advantage of being able to measure aspects of personality functioning that the child may otherwise be less willing or able to reveal, while at the same time offering details about the nonbehavioral level of psychological processes (Leifer et al., 1991; Rasch & Wagner, 1989; Shapiro et al., 1990). For example, attempts have been made to define specific markers in children's human figure and House-Tree-Person drawings, which might serve as reliable indicators of sexual abuse (Cohen & Phelps, 1985; Hibbard, Roghmann, & Hoekelman, 1987). An investigation of the interpretation of childrens' responses to the Hand Test reported that patterns could be detected which distinguished between three groups of sexually abused children, who displayed either severe trauma, neurotic reactions, or no apparent emotional effects (Rasch & Wagner, 1989). An empirical, multidimensional Thematic Apperception Test measure has been developed to assess levels of object relations with psychiatrically disturbed adolescents (Westen, 1991; Westen, Ludolph, Block, Wixom, & Wiss, 1990).

With regard to use of the Rorschach, subsequent to the development and widespread clinical adoption of Exner's comprehensive system of scoring and interpretation (Exner, 1982, 1990, 1991, 1993), many psychometric qualities of the Rorschach have been reported to be at levels roughly comparable to those of the MMPI. Most Rorschach variable scores cannot be assigned with the same certainty as the score for a true/false response inventory. Nevertheless, research reports indicate high interscorer correlations with trained clinicians, and scoring in the Exner Comprehensive System is a reliable and largely objective process. Similarly, Exner's (1991) prescribed schedule for interpretation of the quantitative data yielded by administration of the Rorschach has become highly standardized and systematic.

The Rorschach Inkblot Test has long been used in research studies of the functioning of various diagnostic groups, and more recently it has been used in a growing number of studies attempting to examine the effects of childhood sexual abuse upon the subsequent psychological functioning of both children and adult survivors, and is proving to be increasingly valuable in this area of projective psychodiagnostic research. A recent residential treatment outcome study used the Rorschach to evaluate adolescent personality functioning at admission and after two years of treatment, concluding that the research results indicated the utility of the Rorschach test-retest method of assessing treatment outcome (Abraham, Lepisto, Lewis, Schultz, & Finkelberg, 1994). Of the many available projective instruments, the following comments will focus on two of the most frequently utilized tests, the Rorschach and the Thematic Apperception Test.

1. *The Rorschach Inkblot Test (Rorschach).* The Rorschach Inkblot Test (Rorschach, 1921) consists of a set of 10 specific inkblots. The Rorschach can be administered to subjects from age 5 through adulthood; the average adult takes between 40 and 55 minutes to complete a record, and children average between 30 and 40 minutes. Scoring, computing ratios and percentages, and systematic interpretation of the data can be time-consuming, especially if a subject's number of responses and resulting verbal protocol is lengthy. The Rorschach yields data unique to the individual subject on a number of dimensions, including: affective functioning, interpersonal functioning, self-perception, psychological controls and stress tolerance, and cognitive functioning (including areas related to the intake of information, the interpretation of information, and the quality of thought processes). Specialized constellation configurations yield data regarding severity of depression, suicide potential, and some indicators of specific psychodiagnostic categories. In addition, other researchers have developed experimental scales to broadly estimate the levels of object relations (Urist, 1977) and object representation (Blatt & Lerner, 1983; Fritsch & Holmstrom, 1990; Stuart, Westen, Lohr, Benjamin, Becker, Vurus, & Silk, 1990).

2. *The Thematic Apperception Test (TAT).* The Thematic Apperception Test (Murray, 1943) is comprised of 21 pictures, from which clinicians usually choose 8-10 to administer to subjects 13 years of age and older. The Children's Apperception Test (CAT; Bellak & Bellak,

1949) is available for use with children up to the age of 10 years; some clinicians prefer use of the Roberts Apperception Test for Children (RATC; McArthur & Roberts, 1982), since it can be scored according to an objective scoring system.

Depending upon the particular pictures the clinician chooses to administer, the subject's TAT stories can evoke information about a number of issues or themes, including: general emotional state, attitudes toward authority figures in general, issues related to feelings about performance adequacy or inadequacy, attitudes toward parental figures, interpersonal relationships, intimate relationships, levels of aggression, super-ego development, sexuality, and defense/coping mechanisms.

Although the TAT is one of the top five mentioned assessment tools by clinicians for inclusion in psychological test batteries, its use in research is rare. Despite Bellak's (1954) early efforts to systematize TAT interpretation, it lacks psychometric soundness, in part due both to the variety of pictures chosen for administration to subjects and to the significant influence of clinician subjectivity in interpreting subjects' stories. Nevertheless, there have been some efforts to place interpretation of the TAT on a more empirical base, specifically on experimental research on the TAT and estimates of object relations (Westen, 1991; Westen, Ludolph, Block, Wixom, & Wiss, 1990).

## CONCLUSION

This study surveyed some of the practical and methodological difficulties related to residential treatment outcome research. For example, earlier criticisms of outcome research noted that studies utilized a variety of treatment methods, were often unclear about criteria for measuring improvement, had differing foci (e.g., diagnosis, sample description, disposition, or current level of functioning), and seldom focused clearly upon the actual treatment process.

More recent commentaries have noted the increased importance of funding and fiscal accountability as one of the major goals for the development and implementation of an outcome assessment research program. Recent studies have also noted continuing methodological weaknesses, including: problems in specifying the programmatic components of residential care as clearly defined and measurable treatment interventions; failures to study the milieu in a rigorous manner; and the paucity of residential outcome research presenting clear measurement of actual treatment implementation. Other frequently noted challenges to sound empirical outcome assessment have included purportedly inadequate demographic descriptions of the specific populations in residential treatment settings and the difficulty in selecting valid and reliable formal assessment instruments, related both to demographic indicants of a particular residential setting's population, and to formal outcome measures of treatment effectiveness.

The paper concluded with a survey list of possible outcome assessment instruments, which included descriptions of selected (1) clinical interview schedules, (2) objective rating scales (including global functioning, behavioral, and specialized focus scales), (3) objective personality inventories, and (4) projective tests. The descriptive and comparative listing briefly described each instrument's general structure, intended subject group, stated purpose or goal, psychometrics, and, when applicable, special considerations related to use of the instrument.

## REFERENCES

Abraham, P. P., Lepisto, B. L., Lewis, M. G., Schultz, L., & Finkelberg, S. (1994). An outcome study: Changes in Rorschach variables of adolescents in residential treatment. *Journal of Personality Assessment, 62*(3), 505-514.

Achenbach, T. M. (1991a). *Manual for the Child Behavior Checklist/4-18 and 1991 Profile.* Burlington, Vt.: Univ. of Vermont Department of Psychiatry.

Achenbach, T. M. (1991b). *Manual for the Youth Self-Report and 1991 Profile.* Burlington, Vt.: Univ. of Vermont Department of Psychiatry.

Archer, R. P., Maruish, M. Imhof, E. A., & Piotrowski, C. (1991). Psychological Test Usage with Adolescent Clients: 1990 Survey Findings. *Professional Psychology: Research and Practice, 22*, p. 249.

Bellak, L. (1954). *The T.A.T., C.A.T. and S.A.T. in Clinical Use* (10th Ed.). New York: Grune & Stratton.

_____ & Bellak, S. S. (1949). *Children's Apperception Test (CAT).* Larchmont, N. Y.: C. P. S. Inc.

Belter, R. W., Lipovsky, J. A., & Finch, A. J. (1989). Rorschach egocentricity index and self-concept in children and adolescents. *Journal of Personality Assessment, 53*(4), 783-789.

Blatt, S. J., & Lerner, H. (1983). The psychological assessment of object representation. *Journal of Personality Assessment, 47*, 7-28.

Butcher, J. N., Williams, C. L., Graham, J. R., Archer, R. P., Tellegen, A., Ben-Porath, Y. S., & Kaemmer, B. (1992). *MMPI-A (Minnesota Multiphasic Personality Inventory-Adolescent): Manual for Administration, Scoring, and Interpretation.* Minneapolis, Minn.: University of Minnesota Press.

Cohen, F. W., & Phelps, R. E. (1985). Incest markers in children's artwork. *The Arts in Psychotherapy, 12*, 265-283.

Conners, C. K. (1989). *Manual for Conners' Rating Scales*. North Tonawanda, N.Y.: Multi-Health Systems.

Conoley, J. C., & Kramer, J. J. (1989). *Tenth Mental Measurements Yearbook*. Lincoln, Nebraska: The University of Nebraska Press.

Coopersmith, S. (1987). *Coopersmith Self-Esteem Inventories Manual*. Palo Alto, Cal.: Consulting Psychologists Press.

Curry, John F. (1995). The current status of research in residential treatment. *Residential Treatment for Children & Youth, 12*(3), 1-17.

Dimperio, T. L., Blotcky, M. J., Gossett, J. T., & Doyle, A. H. (1986). The Timberlawn child functioning scale: A preliminary report on reliability and validity. *The Psychiatric Hospital, 17*, 115-120.

Endicott, J., Spitzer, R. L., Fleiss, J. L., & Cohen, J. (1976). The Global Assessment Scale: A procedure for measuring overall severity of psychiatric disturbance. *Archives of General Psychiatry, 33*, 766-771.

Everson, M. D., Hunter, W. M., Runyon, D. K., Edelsohn, G. A., & Coulter, M. L. (1989). Maternal support following disclosure of incest. *American Journal of Orthopsychiatry, 59*, 197-207.

Exner, J. E. (1982). *The Rorschach: A Comprehensive System*. (Vol. 3, 1st Ed.). New York: Wiley.

Exner, J. E. (1990). *A Rorschach Workbook for the Comprehensive System* (3rd Ed.). Asheville, N. C.: Rorschach Workshops.

Exner, J. E. (1991). *The Rorschach: A Comprehensive System* (Vol. 2, 2nd Ed.). New York: Wiley.

Exner, J. E. (1993). *The Rorschach: A Comprehensive System* (Vol. 1, 3rd Ed.). New York: Wiley.

Eyberg, S. (1992). Parent and teacher behavior inventories for the assessment of conduct behaviors in children. In L. VandeCreek & L. G. Ritt (Eds.), *Innovations in Clinical Practice: A Source Book* (Vol. 11). Sarasota, Fl.: Professional Resource Exchange.

Fischer, J., & Corcoran, K. (1994). *Measures for Clinical Practice: A Sourcebook* (vols. 1 and 2, 2nd Ed.). New York: The Free Press.

Friedrich, W. N., & Reams, R. A. (1987). Course of psychological symptoms in sexually abused young children. *Psychotherapy, 24*(2), 160-170.

Fritsch, R. C., & Holmstrom, R. W. (1990). Assessing object representations as a continuous variable: A modification of the concept of the object on the Rorschach scale. *Journal of Personality Assessment, 55* (1&2), 319-334.

Garber, B. (1972). *Follow-up Study of Hospitalized Adolescents*. New York: Brunner/Mazel.

Gossett, J., Lewis, J., & Barnhart, D. (1983). *To Find a Way: The Outcome of Hospital Treatment of Disturbed Adolescents*. New York: Brunner/Mazel.

Hammill, D. D., Brown, L., & Bryant, B. R. (1992). *A Consumer's Guide to Tests in Print* (2nd Ed.). Austin, Texas: Pro-Ed Publishers.

Hartmann, E., Glasser, B., Greenblatt, M., Soloman, & Levinson, D. (1968). *Adolescents in a Mental Hospital*. New York: Grune & Stratton.

Herjanic, B., & Campbell, W. (1977). Differentiating psychiatrically disturbed children on the basis of a structured interview. *Journal of Abnormal Child Psychology, 51*, 127-134.

Hibbard, R. A., Roghmann, K., & Hoekelman, R. A. (1987). Genitalia in children's drawings: An association with sexual abuse. *Pediatrics, 79*(1), 129-137.

Hodges, K., Kline, S., Fitch, P., McKnew, D., & Cytryn, L. (1981). The Child Assessment Schedule: A diagnostic interview for research and clinical use. Washington, D.C.: American Psychological Association.

Jesness, D. F. (1984). *Jesness Behavior Checklist Manual.* Palo Alto, Cal.: Consulting Psychologists Press.

Jesness, D. F. (1988). *Jesness Inventory Manual.* Palo Alto, Cal.: Consulting Psychologists Press.

Kazdin, A. E., French, H. H., & Unis, A. S. (1983). Child, mother and father evaluations of depression in psychiatric inpatient children. *Journal of Abnormal Child Psychology, 11*, 167-180.

Keyser, D. J., & Sweetland, R. C. (Eds.) (1985). *Test Critiques* (vol. 1). Kansas City, Mo.: Test Corporation of America.

Klinge, V., Piggot, L., Knitter, E., & O'Donnell, A. (1986). A follow-up study of psychiatrically hospitalized adolescents. *Adolescence, 83*, 697-701.

Leifer, M., Shapiro, J. P., Martone, M. W., & Kassem, L. (1991). Rorschach assessment of psychological functioning in sexually abused girls. *Journal of Personality Assessment, 56*(1), 14-28.

MacArthur, D. S., & Roberts, G. E. (1982). *Roberts Apperception Test for Children.* Los Angeles, Cal.: Western Psychological Services.

McGlashan, T. H., & Keats, C. J. (1989). *Schizophrenia: Treatment Process and Outcome.* Washington, D. C.: American Psychiatric Press, Inc.

McLeer, S. V., Deblinger, E., Atkins, M. S., Foa, E. B., & Ralphe, D. L. (1988). Post-traumatic stress disorder in sexually abused children. *Journal of the Academy of Child and Adolescent Psychiatry, 27*(5), 650-654.

Miller, L. C. (1984). *Louisville Behavior Checklist Manual.* Los Angeles, Cal.: Western Psychological Services.

Millon, T., Green, C. J., & Meagher, R. B. (1982). *Millon Adolescent Personality Inventory Manual.* Minneapolis, Minn.: National Computer Systems.

Mitchell, J. V., Jr. (1983). *Tests in Print III: An Index to Tests, Test Reviews, and the Literature on Specific Tests.* Lincoln, Nebraska: Buros Institute of Mental Measurements, University of Nebraska-Lincoln.

Mordock, J. B. (in press). The search for an identity: A call for observational-inductive research methods in residential treatment. *Residential Treatment for Children & Youth.*

Moretti, M. M., Fine, S., Haley, G., & Marriage, K. (1985). Childhood and adolescent depression: Child-report versus parent-report information. *Journal of the American Academy of Child Psychiatry, 24*, 298-302.

Murray, H. A. (1943). *Thematic Apperception Test Manual.* Cambridge, Mass.: Harvard University Press.

Naglieri, J. A., LeBuffe, P. A., & Pfeiffer, S. I. (1994). *Devereux Scales of Psychopathology.* San Antonio, Tx.: The Psychological Corporation.

Parker, K. C. H., Hanson, R. K., & Hunsley, J. (1988). MMPI, Rorschach, and WAIS: A meta-analytic comparison of reliability, stability, and validity. *The Psychological Bulletin, 103*, 367-373.

Pfeiffer, S. I., Burd, S., and Wright, A. (1992). Clinicians and research: Recurring obstacles and some possible solutions. *Journal of Clinical Psychology, 48*(1), 140-145.

Pfeiffer, S. I., Soldivera, S., & Norton, J. (1992). *A Consumer's Guide to Mental Health Treatment Outcome Measures.* Devon, Pa.: The Devereux Institute of Clinical Training & Research.

Piers, E. V. (1984). *Piers-Harris Children's Self-Concept Scale Revised Manual.* Los Angeles, Cal.: Western Psychological Services.

Prentice-Dunn, S., & Lyman, R. D. (1989). In R. D. Lyman, S. Prentice-Dunn, & S. Gabel (Eds.), *Residential and Inpatient Treatment of Children and Adolescents.* New York: Plenum Press.

Rasch, M. A., & Wagner, E. E. (1989). Initial psychological effects of sexual abuse on female children as reflected in the hand test. *Journal of Personality Assessment, 54*(4), 761-769.

Robinson, J. P., Shaver, P. R., & Wrightsman, L. S. (1991). *Measures of Personality and Social Psychological Attitudes.* New York: Academic Press.

Roid, G. H., & Fitts, W. H. (1988). *Tennessee Self-Concept Scale-Revised Manual.* Los Angeles, Cal.: Western Psychological Services.

Rorschach, H. (1921). *Psychodiagnostics.* (Hans Huber Verlag, Transl. 1942). Bern: Bircher.

Shaffer, D., Gould, M. S., Brasie, J., Ambrosini, P., Fisher, P., Bird, H., & Aluwahilia, S. (1983). A children's global assessment scale (CGAS). *Archives of General Psychiatry, 40*, 1228-1231.

Shapiro, J. P., Leifer, M., Martone, M. W., & Kassem, L. (1990). Multimethod assessment of depression in sexually abused girls. *Journal of Personality Assessment 55*(1&2), 234-248.

Spitzer, R. L., Endicott, J. L., & Cohen, J. (1970). Psychiatric Status Schedule: A technique for evaluating psychopathology and impairment in role functioning. *Archives of General Psychiatry, 23*, 41-55.

Stuart, J., Westen, D., Lohr, N., Benjamin, J., Becker, S., Vorus, N. & Silk, K. (1990). Object relations in borderlines, depressives, and normals: An examination of human responses on the Rorschach. *Journal of Personality Assessment, 55*(1&2), 296-318.

Sweetland, R. C., & Keyser, D. J. (1991). *Tests: A Comprehensive Reference for Assessment in Psychology, Education and Business* (3rd Ed.). Austin, Texas: Pro-Ed Publishers.

Tong, L., Oates, K., & McDowell, M. (1987). Personality development following sexual abuse. *Child Abuse & Neglect, 11*, 371-383.

Urist, J. (1977). The Rorschach test and the assessment of object relations. *Journal of Personality Assessment, 41*, 3-9.

Vermillion, J. M., & Pfeiffer, S. I. (1993). Treatment outcome and continuous quality improvement: Two aspects of program evaluation. *The Psychiatric Hospital, 24*(1/2), 9-14.

Wallerstein, R. S. (1986). *Forty-Two Lives in Treatment: A Study of Psychoanalysis and Psychotherapy.* New York: Guilford Press.

Westen, D. (1991). Clinical assessment of object relations using the TAT. *Journal of Personality Assessment, 56*(1), 56-74.

Westen, D., Ludolph, P., Block, J., Wixom, J., & Wiss, F. C. (1990). Developmental history and object relations in psychiatrically disturbed adolescent girls. *American Journal of Psychiatry, 147*(8), 1061-1068.

Whittaker, J. K., Overstreet, E. J., Grasso, A., Tripodi, T., & Boylan, F. (1988). Multiple indicators of success in residential youth care and treatment. *American Journal of Orthopsychiatry, 58*(1), 143-147.

Wilson, D., & Lyman, R. (1983). Residential treatment of emotionally disturbed children. In C. Walker & M. Roberts (Eds.), *Handbook of Clinical Child Psychology.* New York: Wiley.

# Implementing
# an Outcome Assessment Project:
# Logistical, Practical,
# and Ethical Considerations

Steven I. Pfeiffer, Phd, ABPP
Susan Shott, EdM

**SUMMARY.** In today's healthcare environment, there is a rapidly growing demand for accountability. With this pressure to verify treatment effectiveness, outcome measures are being used to provide objective evidence that the care being delivered is appropriate, satisfactory, effective, and cost-efficient. In addition to important conceptual, methodological, and psychometric factors, there are a number of pragmatic considerations involved in a successful outcome assessment project. This article will examine eight such considerations: setting realistic goals; assembling a project team, enlisting commitments of staff, agency, clients and funding sources; managing the logistics of the project; handling of the data; using the results most effectively; budgeting for the project; and attending to ethical issues. *[Article copies available from The Haworth Document Delivery Service: 1-800-342-9678. E-mail address: getinfo@haworth.com]*

Steven I. Pfeiffer is Director of Behavioral Health, Genesis Health Ventures, and Professor of Psychology in Psychiatry, University of Pennsylvania School of Medicine. Susan Shott is affiliated with Devereux Institute of Clinical Training & Research.

Steven I. Pfeiffer may be written at Genesis Health Ventures, Managed Care Division, 312 West State Street, Kennett Square, PA 19348.

[Haworth co-indexing entry note]: "Implementing an Outcome Assessment Project: Logistical, Practical, and Ethical Considerations." Pfeiffer, Steven I., and Susan Shott. Co-published simultaneously in *Residential Treatment for Children & Youth* (The Haworth Press, Inc.) Vol. 13, No. 4, 1996, pp. 71-81; and: *Outcome Assessment in Residential Treatment* (ed: Steven I. Pfeiffer) The Haworth Press, Inc., 1996, pp. 71-81. Single or multiple copies of this article are available from The Haworth Document Delivery Service [1-800-342-9678, 9:00 a.m. - 5:00 p.m. (EST). E-mail address: getinfo@haworth.com].

## INTRODUCTION

Because residential treatment and psychiatric hospitalization are under increasing attack (e.g., Henggeler, 1994), it is essential for providers of mental healthcare services in campus-based settings to demonstrate the effectiveness of the therapeutic services that they provide. These mental healthcare providers are increasingly caught between the push to contain costs and the need to prove–and improve–both effectiveness and quality of their services (Carbine, M., 1992). In response, various stakeholders–including professional peer groups, regulatory organizations, and market forces–are using outcome measures to verify treatment effectiveness.

Treatment outcome studies evaluate the impact a treatment program has on a client's clinical status and psychosocial functioning and provide an objective basis for the consumer's and purchaser's evaluation of the quality of care provided. They also provide an opportunity to better understand which factors predict successful outcome, identify the types of clients for whom a given treatment is likely to be most effective, and generate statistical baselines for the success of various planned interventions (Vermillion & Pfeiffer, 1990).

The successful implementation of an outcomes assessment project in a residential treatment facility is no simple undertaking. As discussed by the preceding authors, important theoretical, conceptual, methodological, and psychometric factors need to be considered. To ensure a successful outcomes assessment project, however, a number of pragmatic considerations are equally important. This article will discuss the following eight considerations: setting realistic goals; enlisting the commitment of staff, agency, clients, and funding sources; managing the logistics of the project; securing technical assistance; handling the data; using the results most effectively; budgeting for the project; and attending to ethical issues.

## SETTING REALISTIC GOALS

### Modest Scope

In planning outcome assessment projects, it is prudent to initially "think small" and look toward launching a pilot project of modest scope. Our experience at Devereux has led us to start with comparatively small, straightforward projects in order to assess feasibility, organizational readiness, and receptivity. Only after we have experienced success with a small scale, pilot project do we encourage an iterative process of revising, expanding, and elaborating the protocol into a more comprehensive and sophisticated outcome assessment project.

## ASSEMBLING A PROJECT TEAM

The project team has the responsibility for obtaining consensus on the purpose of the project and helping to frame the assessment questions (see Pratt & Moreland in this issue). We have found that enlisting a group of clinicians interested in outcome assessment–or at least comfortable with the philosophy of psychological measurement and accountability–assists in setting realistic and accomplishable goals. Davies, Doyle, Lansky et al. (1994) suggest that a project team include a project coordinator who serves as task manager, change agent, and liaison between clinical staff and outcomes assessment technical staff. At Devereux, project teams have played a key role in determining the feasibility of the proposed outcomes assessment, ensuring that the agency is not prematurely taking on too difficult of a project.

We have seen project teams help orchestrate outcome assessment projects through developmental stages of increasing complexity and sophistication. For example:

- small scale to larger scale,
- pilot to demonstration to full agency adoption/integration,
- time-limited to ongoing,
- simple (e.g., one-group posttest only) to more complex design (e.g., non-equivalent comparison group pretest-posttest design or multiple-series design).

Project teams serve a valuable role not only in assuring the feasibility of an outcome assessment protocol, but also in striking a balance between methodological rigor and pragmatic considerations. For example, a particular structured clinical interview might be an excellent instrument of choice based on reliability, validity, and frequency that is cited in the professional literature (e.g., SCID; Spitzer, Williams, Gibbon, & First, 1990). The project team, however, might find that the complexity of the instrument, as well as the amount of training and time required for administration and scoring, make it less attractive than other less complex or costly measures (see the article by Green and Newman in this volume).

## ENLISTING THE COMMITMENT OF STAFF, AGENCY, CLIENTS AND FUNDING SOURCES

### Staff and Agency Buy-In

An outcome assessment project requires the support of the highest levels of the organization. The agency's leaders need to communicate a clear and strong message of endorsement, conveying the importance of undertaking outcome assessment to ensure improved services and continuous learning (Deming, 1986; Senge, 1990; Vermillion & Pfeiffer, 1990). As discussed earlier, one role of the project team is to set realistic and accomplishable goals. Equally important is for the team to illustrate to the organization the value-added in undertaking an outcome assessment project. We, at Devereux, have found that agency buy-in is greatly facilitated when one team member, typically a clinician, serves as "champion" of the project. Since it is not unreasonable to experience initial staff resistance, the champion can serve a critical function in promoting staff enthusiasm and even shared ownership of the various components of the project (e.g., selecting instruments, collecting data, and explaining the purpose of the study to clients and parents). As a project matures developmentally to a "maintenance" stage, less effort is demanded of the champion and team to promote the value-added to the organization of the project (Davies et al., 1994).

## Client and Family Commitment

Equally important to the success of an outcome assessment project is the interest and commitment of the clients and family members. Our experience has led us to enlist client and parent involvement at the time of admissions. It is helpful to explain the purpose of the project, what will be expected of the client and the parents, and the benefits that will accrue as the agency examines the findings of the outcome project. Informational newsletters and presentations by project team members during Family Day visits are but two ways of educating clients and parents on the value of their participation in the data collection process. Compensation in the form of a nominal stipend ($10.00-$20.00) or a gift coupon (e.g., $5.00 toward a meal at McDonald's or Burger King) has also been used by applied researchers to boost the subject response rate, and can be a beneficial, if costly, incentive.

It is particularly challenging to procure a high rate of participation after clients have been discharged from the facility. For example, in a methodology review of 32 outcome studies published since 1975, we found that subject attrition was a major problem at time of follow-up assessment. Twenty-seven percent of the studies reported 51% to 75% compliance, and 10% of the studies reported a less than 51% respondent rate (Pfeiffer, 1989). Strategies to further client and parent commitment early on in the treatment process will bear rich dividends when the project team attempts to contact the family post-discharge to enlist their continued participation. Keeping a record of the names, addresses, and telephone numbers of contact persons is critical to retaining a high rate of participation at time of follow-up. One tactic that we have found helpful is routinely sending out holiday and birthday cards to former clients, in part as a means of keeping track of where they are living in the community.

## MANAGING THE LOGISTICS OF THE PROJECT

As discussed in the preceding sections, the project team has to determine the scope of the outcome assessment and decide upon what type of outcome constructs to measure (e.g., reduction in symptomatology, improvement in psychosocial or vocational functioning, enhancement in client satisfaction or quality of life). As Green and Newman so aptly address in their article, the project team also needs to decide upon a best set of instruments to measure the targeted outcome constructs.

Management of the logistics of the project is critical to ensure that the data is collected in a timely, reliable, and unobtrusive fashion consistent with the work flow and organization of the setting (Davies et al., 1994). Key issues that need to be considered include:

- *Who* will collect *which* data?
- *When* will the data be collected?
- *Where* will the data be collected?
- *How often* will *which* data be collected?
- *Who* will enter the data into a database?

Fully appreciating that problems will and do occur, we have found five strategies that help the project team effectively manage the logistics of the outcome assessment. First, develop a *flow chart* that provides a pictorial representation showing all of the steps of the outcome assessment process. Second, devise a *tracking system* and automatic *"tickler" system* to prompt and help maintain protocol integrity.

Third, construct an *operations manual* that "concretizes" all important aspects of the outcome assessment project. We have found that diagrams, tables, figures, and charts all help to identify the various steps in each process of the outcome assessment. These visual aids make it easier for staff to fully understand the project, and therefore foster greater consistency and adherence to the specific requirements of the protocol. Fourth, looking ahead to how the data will ultimately be used and by whom, it is advisable to formulate a *utilization plan*. This point also bears relevance to the issue of ethics, which is addressed in a subsequent section of this article.

The fifth strategy is to provide for *staff training*. Agency personnel will require in-service training to understand the rationale for undertaking treatment outcome at a residential facility. Training will also help staff understand how treatment outcome complements continuous quality improvement (Batalden et al., 1994; Berwick, 1989; Vermillion & Pfeiffer, 1990) and exemplifies a learning organization (Senge, 1990). In addition to providing new knowledge, staff training is important to provide new skills critical to the success of a treatment outcome project–computer literacy and precision in using the outcome instruments, to name but two.

## SECURING TECHNICAL ASSISTANCE

Most organizations will find that even a small scale, pilot outcome assessment project is complex enough to require the support of a consultant. Technical assistance is usually required in one or more of the following areas:

• Helping the project team define the outcomes and select the outcome measures,
• Developing an automated system to store the data; guiding the team in selecting software packages,
• Recommending a format to enter the data; determining the correct statistical program to analyze the data, and
• Designing a report format to present the findings.

Although it is by no means imperative to secure external technical assistance, consultants can prove invaluable in supporting areas of technical complexity.

## HANDLING THE DATA

### Data Entry

Three questions the project team faces when planning data entry into a database are: (1) Who is responsible for performing the data entry function? (2) Should the data be entered in "real time" or can it be delayed? (3) Will the data entry be manual or automated? (Davies et al., 1994).

Our experience at Devereux has led us to recommend a decentralized ownership of the data entry process, which helps ensure that no duplicate data entry occurs. We have found that it is easier and less expensive for staff to delay data entry until a number of completed client forms can be entered in batch configuration. We initially felt that real-time data entry would be beneficial in providing immediate feedback to clinicians; however, our various project teams quickly discovered that it is logistically more practical and fiscally less costly to delay entry until a sizable number of completed forms were available for batch entry.

Most residential facilities are entering data manually, which requires minimal staff training and less costly hardware. However, computer-based assessment is a rapidly growing field, and large behavioral healthcare agencies are beginning to adopt automated assessment and tracking systems with positive results (e.g., Vieweg & DiFranco, 1995). "Cutting edge" technology in automated data entry includes scanners or "optimal mark readers" and computer "touchscreens." However, most of the newly emerging technology is expensive, requires the client to be computer literate, and is not yet designed for use by children or adolescents.

### Data Analysis

The project team must also decide how they want the data analyzed. Two principles guiding this decision are the purpose of the outcome assessment and the projected use of the data.

Data analysis can range from simple aggregate descriptive information to highly sophisticated inferential statistical queries. For example, we recently performed a series of inferential statistical analyses on a data set to better understand the relative influence of a series of predictor and mediating variables on the outcome of a group of adolescents in a short-term facility.

## USING THE RESULTS MOST EFFICIENTLY

To be most useful, outcome assessment projects should be intimately linked to continuous quality improvement (CQI) efforts. Outcome assessment and CQI are complementary because both focus on assessing client programs and providing useful and reliable data to help enhance program effectiveness. The foundations of CQI are assessment and problem-solving, and improvement opportunities are identified through quality assessment. The quality of clinical services continues to be assessed through clinical indicator data based on outcomes of care (Vermillion & Pfeiffer, 1990).

Outcome data can be used by the project team to gain a more accurate and comprehensive understanding of the process related to client care, and in this way it becomes a vital tool on the path toward quality improvement. The measurement of outcomes is necessary, but not sufficient, to improve the quality of care. Improvement in outcomes requires that specific changes be instituted in the client care process. These changes are guided by the team's use of outcome data to identify variations in processes that may be contributing to the obtained outcomes. Batalden et al. (1994) offer the apt analogy, "telling a baseball player about his batting average (or a surgeon about his coronary artery bypass graft mortality rate) is a necessary but insufficient step toward improvement. Results produced by complex systems can be improved predictably only by understanding how each major process in the system affects the results and continually improves each process" (p. 169).

## BUDGETING FOR THE PROJECT

The project team needs to be realistic in estimating the cost of initiating outcome assessment. It has been our experience that the cost generally exceeds the projected budgeted expenses, particularly with costs attributed to start-up of a project.

We recommend that the team estimate costs for each component of the project, including the following line items:

- personnel (percent of effort on the project)
- travel reimbursement
- supplies (test materials, record forms, file cabinets, etc.)
- copying, printing, mailing
- telephone
- equipment (computer, software, printer, etc.)
- compensation to participants
- consultant costs.

## ETHICAL ISSUES

Outcome assessment is considered by many to be a form of research, which imposes ethical considerations and obligations on the residential treatment center.

For example, the following questions can be expected to be raised when undertaking a treatment outcome project:

- Does the project team have to develop special consent forms and obtain informed consent?
- Should the outcome assessment data be filed in the client's clinical record or be kept in a separate file?
- Does the agency need to develop a privacy protection policy similar to a policy that stipulates the need to assess the merits of proposed research and the individuals from whom approval must be obtained?
- Could contact with discharged clients be viewed as intrusive or a violation of their privacy or confidentiality?
- Does the agency have an obligation to advise clients and parents that the facility is engaged in outcome assessment "research" that may affect the client's care or treatment?

These and many other related questions make it imperative for the project team to consider the ethical implications of the outcome assessment.

## Informed Consent

Informed consent is predicated on the principle of providing persons with information that is relevant to their decision of whether or not to participate in the outcome assessment project. The client, and his/her parent or guardian if they are a minor, should be provided with explicit and complete information about the study. Information should include: (1) the purposes of the project, (2) how subjects are being recruited, (3) what their participation will involve, and for how long, (4) the probability and magnitude of harm and benefit to participation, (5) assurances that participation is voluntary, (6) protection of confidentiality and (7) names and affiliations of the members of the project team who are available to answer questions or provide further information.

## Privacy and Confidentiality

The residential treatment agency has the responsibility to respect the privacy of clients and their families by maintaining confidentiality of personal information. Confidentiality protects persons from potential adverse consequences that may occur if personal information is disclosed.

Strategies for protecting confidentiality of clients involved in an outcome assessment project include:

- Limiting access to the outcome data,
- Coding data to protect the identity of clients,

- Storing the data in a locked and secure file cabinet,
- Marking all data and project team documents as confidential,
- Limiting the number of copies of project team reports, and collecting such documents at the close of team meetings,
- Destroying the data after a specified time period,
- Assuring that individual clients cannot be identified if the findings are published, and
- Carefully controlling all client and family contacts.


## CONCLUSION

Outcome assessment studies are invaluable tools to help residential treatment centers evaluate the impact of their therapeutic programs and as a means of complementing CQI efforts. Undertaking outcome assessment requires attention to a number of pragmatic considerations, as well as conceptual, methodological, and psychometric factors, to ensure a successful project.

This paper has addressed eight such considerations: setting realistic goals; enlisting commitments of staff, agency, clients, and funding sources; project management; securing technical assistance; handling of the data; using the results most effectively; budgeting for the project; and dealing with the ethical issues. We believe that thoughtfully conceived outcome assessment protocols will bear rich dividends to the agency, staff, and clients and families that we serve.


## REFERENCES

Batalden, P.B., Nelson, E.C., & Roberts, J.S. (1994). Linking outcomes measurement to continual improvement. *Journal for Quality Improvement, 20(4)*, 167-180.

Berwick, D.M. (1989). Sounding board: Continuous improvement as an ideal in healthcare. *New England Journal of Medicine, 320*, 53.

Carbine, M. (Ed.)(1992). Using outcome measures in mental health care. *PhysicianMANAGER*, 3(10), 1,6-8.

Davies, A.R., Doyle, M.A.T., Lansky, D., Rutt, W., Stevic, M.O., & Doyle, J.B. (1994). Outcomes assessment in clinical settings: A consensus statement on principles and best practices in project management. *Journal for Quality Improvement, 20*(1), 6-16.

Deming, W.E. (1986). *Out of Crisis*. Cambridge, MA: Massachusetts Institute of Technology Press.

Henggeler, S.W. (Ed.)(1994). Task force report on innovative models of mental health services for children, adolescents, and their families. *Journal of Clinical Child Psychology, 23* (Supplement), 1-62.

Pfeiffer, S.I. (1989). Follow-up of children and adolescents treatment in psychiatric facilities: A methodology review. *The Psychiatric Hospital, 20(1)*, 15-20.

Senge, P.M. (1990). *The Fifth Discipline: The art and practice of the learning organization*. New York: Doubleday.

Spitzer, R.L., Williams, J.B.W., Gibbon, M., & First, M.B. (1990). *SCID: Structured Clinical Interview for DSM-III-R*. Washington, DC: American Psychiatric Press, Inc.

Vermillion, J.M., & Pfeiffer, S.I. (1990). Treatment outcome and continuous quality improvement: Two aspects of program evaluation. *The Psychiatric Hospital, 24(12)*, 9-14.

Vieweg, B.W., & DiFranco, B. (1995). The use of automated assessment with seriously mentally ill clients. *Behavioral Healthcare Tomorrow, Jan/Feb*, 37-41.

# Measuring Outcomes
# in Residential Treatment
# with the Devereux Scales
# of Mental Disorders

Paul A. Lebuffe, MA
Steven I. Pfeiffer, PhD, ABPP

**SUMMARY.** The Devereux Scales of Mental Disorders is unique among child and adolescent behavior rating scales in that it provides an explicit methodology for evaluating treatment outcome. The approach utilizes a dual criterion of statistically reliable and clinically meaningful change which is used to operationally define five clinical outcomes: Optimal, Very Favorable, Favorable, Equivocal and Negative. The use of the Devereux Scales of Mental Disorders in evaluating treatment outcome at both the individual client and unit levels is presented. It is hoped that this methodology will assist mental health professionals in responding to the increasing demands for accountability and demonstrated efficacy in child and adolescent treatment. *[Article copies available from The Haworth Document Delivery Service: 1-800-342-9678. E-mail address: getinfo@haworth.com]*

Twenty-five years ago, Bednar and Shapiro (1970) surveyed over 16,000 psychiatrists and psychologists and reported that only 85 individu-

Paul A. Lebuffe is affiliated with the Institute of Clinical Training and Research, The Devereux Foundation, Devon, PA. Steven I. Pfeiffer is affiliated with Genesis Health Ventures, Kennett Square, PA.

[Haworth co-indexing entry note]: "Measuring Outcomes in Residential Treatment with the Devereux Scales of Mental Disorders." Lebuffe, Paul A., and Steven I. Pfeiffer. Co-published simultaneously in *Residential Treatment for Children & Youth* (The Haworth Press, Inc.) Vol. 13, No. 4, 1996, pp. 83-91; and: *Outcome Assessment in Residential Treatment* (ed: Steven I. Pfeiffer) The Haworth Press, Inc., 1996, pp. 83-91. Single or multiple copies of this article are available from The Haworth Document Delivery Service [1-800-342-9678, 9:00 a.m. - 5:00 p.m. (EST). E-mail address: getinfo@haworth.com].

*83*

als (0.5%) were interested in becoming involved in a psychotherapy process outcome project. That few practicing psychologists engage in applied research or consider it to be part of their job was confirmed in a more recent series of studies (Pfeiffer, 1992; Pfeiffer, Burd, & Wright, 1992). Less than five years later, this situation is rapidly changing as professionals involved in child and adolescent mental health treatment are being increasingly challenged to document the effectiveness of their interventions.

The professional and market forces contributing to the growing expectation that practitioners should objectively document the effectiveness of their therapeutic practices has been described by Pratt and Moreland in this volume and in a number of other sources (Linder, 1991; Mirin & Namerow, 1991; O'Leary, 1993) and due to space limitation will not be reviewed here. Suffice it to say that clinicians practicing in residential settings find themselves facing a dilemma; they are increasingly expected to participate in and even direct treatment outcome studies while they often feel that they lack the time, the financial support, the support staff, the physical resources, and perhaps even the interest to conduct applied research studies (Pfeiffer, Burd, & Wright, 1992). The Devereux Scales of Mental Disorders (Naglieri, LeBuffe & Pfeiffer, 1994) were developed in part to address this need for a straightforward, economical, clinically useful and procedurally sound measure to assess treatment outcome in residential and other mental health treatment settings.

## THE DEVEREUX SCALES OF MENTAL DISORDERS

The Devereux Scales of Mental Disorders (DSMD) is a measure of behaviors related to psychopathology in children and adolescents. The content of the scale is derived primarily from the diagnostic criteria of the *Diagnostic and Statistical Manual of the American Psychiatric Association, Fourth Edition (DSM-IV)* (American Psychiatric Association, 1994) and reflects the full range of psychopathology including severely disturbed behaviors such as fire-setting, self-stimulatory and self-abusive behaviors, and hurting or torturing animals.

The 110-item child form (ages 5-12) and the 111-item adolescent form (ages 13-18) can be completed by parents, teachers, or other adults who fill these roles who have at least a sixth-grade reading level. A five point scale ranging from "never" to "very frequently" is used to indicate how often the specific behavior was observed during the previous four weeks. Separate norms are provided for parent and teacher raters and for the gender of the individual being rated. The DSMD takes about fifteen minutes for the rater to complete and about ten minutes to score.

The DSMD provides 10 behavioral indices: a Total Scale score, three second-order composite scores, and six first-order factorially-derived scale scores. The scores are arranged hierarchically with the Total Scale comprised of the three composites each of which is based on two first-order scales (see Figure 1). The Externalizing Composite is comprised of the Conduct and Attention Scales at the child age level and the Conduct and Delinquency Scales at the adolescent age level. For all ages, the Internalizing Composite is based on the Anxiety and Depression Scales, and the Critical Pathology Composite is comprised of the Autism and Acute Problems Scales. $T$ scores ($M = 50$, $SD = 10$) are used in reporting all scale scores with higher scores reflecting more severe and/or pervasive psychopathology. Information on scale development, standardization, reliability and validity are presented in the DSMD manual.

FIGURE 1. Devereux Scale of Mental Disorders Scale Hierarchy.

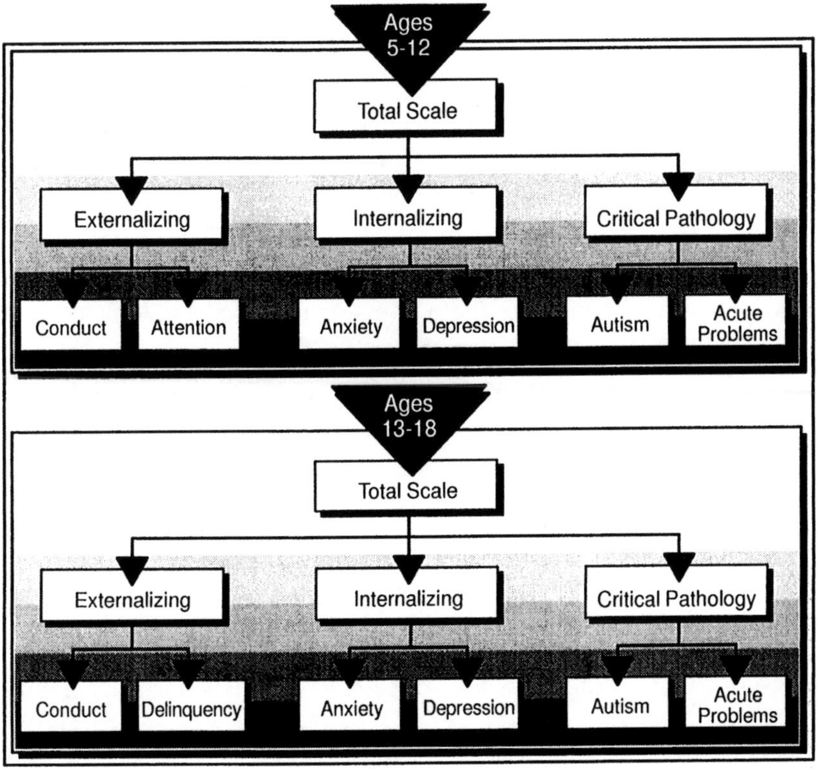

## USE OF THE DSMD IN TREATMENT OUTCOME RESEARCH

The DSMD is unique among behavior rating scales in that it provides an explicit methodology for its use as a treatment outcome measure. The approach is based on a dual criterion of statistically significant (i.e., reliable) and clinically meaningful change. The first aspect of this dual criterion ensures that the change in $T$ scores exceeds that which would be expected by chance and regression effects. In other words, that the difference in pretest-posttest scores reflects "real differences as opposed to ones that are illusory, questionable or unreliable" (Jacobsen & Truax, 1991, p. 12). The second aspect of the dual criterion concerns the social validity or "real-life" meaning of the reported change in the client's behavior.

The DSMD operationalizes the first aspect of the dual criterion by providing tables in the manual which specify a range of posttest scores an individual must exceed in order for the change from a given pretest score to be deemed statistically significant. These ranges were constructed utilizing the standard error of prediction ($SEp$) which accounts for both measurement error and regression effects (Atkinson, 1991; Lord & Novick, 1968).

To illustrate the use of the $SEp$, suppose an adolescent male was rated by a parent at the beginning of treatment and obtained a Total Scale score of 70. The posttest confidence range of 66 to 73 was determined by consulting the appropriate table in the DSMD manual. Posttest scores that exceed this confidence range (greater than 73 in this example) would indicate reliable deterioration in the adolescent's behavior. Conversely, scores below the confidence range (less than 66 in this example) would indicate reliable improvement. Posttest scores that fall within the interval would represent nothing more than chance variation.

Once it has been determined that statistically reliable change has occurred, the second aspect of the dual criterion, the clinical meaningfulness of the change, is determined. As Jacobsen and Truax (1991) noted, clinical meaningfulness has "something to do with the return to normal functioning," which can be conceptualized as "clients entering therapy as part of a dysfunctional population and . . . departing from therapy as no longer belonging to that population" (p. 13). Jacobsen and Truax recommended that a posttest score that places the "client closer to the mean of the functional population than . . . the mean of the dysfunctional population" (p. 13) be used as an operational definition of clinical meaningfulness. As explained in the criterion validity section of the DSMD manual, a Total Scale score of 60 is the best cut-score for differentiating non-clinical from clinical cases. Therefore, when statistically reliable change has occurred, a posttest score of less than 60 is considered to represent clinically meaning-ful change in that it indicates that the client's behavior was perceived as more similar to "normal" individuals than to other individuals with psy-chiatric disorders.

### Operationalizing Clinical Outcomes

We conceptualize five clinical outcomes using the DSMD as a measure of treatment effectiveness. The first three outcomes require statistically reliable improvement in the client's behavior as determined by the *SEp*, and are considered positive outcomes.

"Optimal" outcomes are defined by posttest *T* scores less than 60 and represent behavior that is indistinguishable from non-referred, "normal" individuals. Outcomes in this category meet the dual criterion of statisti-cally reliable and clinically meaningful change.

"Very Favorable" outcomes are defined by posttest scores ranging from 60-69. Although they have not satisfied the strict criterion of clinical-ly meaningful change as defined by Jacobsen and Truax, preliminary evidence indicates that scores in this range are characteristic of individuals in active treatment whose overt behavioral pathology has been stabilized.

"Favorable" outcomes are defined by posttest *T* scores of 70 or above. These elevated outcome scores indicate the continued presence of psycho-pathology. However, because reliable improvement was noted in the cli-ent's behavior since the initial assessment, we consider this to be a positive outcome.

Posttest scores that fall within the confidence interval reflect "Equivo-cal" outcomes because there is no evidence that the client has either appreciably improved or deteriorated. Finally, posttest scores that fall above the confidence interval indicate behavioral deterioration and are characterized as "Negative" clinical outcomes.

We have described how the dual criterion of statistically reliable and clinically meaningful change can be applied to the Total Scale Score, the most reliable and general index on the DSMD. The same approach can be used to examine score changes in the three DSMD composites (Externaliz-ing, Internalizing and Critical Pathology) and the six first-order scales (Conduct, Attention/Delinquency, Anxiety, Depression, Autism and Acute Problems). Pretest-posttest comparisons tables are provided in the DSMD manual for each composite and scale and specify the posttest confidence range for each pretest score. The determination of the clinical significance of changes at the composite or scale score level follows the same logic and uses the same operational definitions of clinical outcome as used with the Total Scale score. Analysis at these more detailed levels supplements the

Total Scale score comparisons and provides additional information on the specific effects of therapeutic interventions.

### Program Evaluation with the DSMD

Clinical outcome data from a number of clients can be combined to evaluate treatment programs or units of service. For example, outcomes for 48 successive discharges from a short-term psychiatric hospital unit at Devereux were evaluated using the approach described above. These clients had a wide range of severe psychiatric disorders and ranged in age from 5 to 20 ($M = 12.5$, $SD = 3.9$). Sixty percent of the sample were male and 40% female. Length of stay varied from 3 to 137 days ($M = 24$, $SD = 26$).

Table 1 presents the aggregated outcomes for this sample and indicates that, based on the Total Scale score, 60% of the clients had a positive outcome (21% Optimal, 25% Very Favorable, and 14% Favorable). Outcomes were judged equivocal for 17% and negative for 23% of the patients.

The DSMD also provides a means of generating and testing hypotheses related to the prediction of clinical course by contrasting the characteristics of the clients that comprise the various clinical outcome groups. For instance, Table 2 presents the percentages of clients in the Optimal and Negative Outcome groups who had significant intraindividual elevations

TABLE 1. Clinical Outcomes for Hospital Sample (n = 48)

| Outcome | % of Clients |
|---|---|
| Positive | |
| "Optimal" - Posttest ≤ 59 | 21 |
| "Very Favorable" - Posttest = 60-69 | 25 |
| "Favorable" - Posttest ≥ 70 | 14 |
| Equivocal | 17 |
| Negative | 23 |
| Total | 100 |

TABLE 2. Intraindividual Scale Elevations for "Optimal" and "Negative" Outcomes

| | Outcome | |
|---|---|---|
| Scale | Optimal (n = 10) | Negative (n = 11) |
| Conduct | 20 | 36 |
| Attention/Delinquency | 20 | 55 |
| Anxiety | 20 | 9 |
| Depression | 60 | 18 |
| Autism | 20 | 9 |
| Acute Problems | 20 | 18 |

Note. The values represent the percent of clients with an intraindividual elevation on the indicated scale.

on each of the six DSMD Scales at admission. Intraindividual analysis compares the six individual scale scores to the mean scale score for each client. An intraindividual scale elevation indicates that the scale score was significantly higher than the average scale score for that client, and thereby may indicate an area of particular concern for that individual. Because an individual can have more than one significant intraindividual scale elevation, the columns in Table 2 sum to more than 100%.

Inspection of Table 2 indicates that 60% of the clients comprising the Optimal Outcome group but only 18% of the clients in the Negative Outcome group had significant elevations on the Depression Scale at admission. In contrast, the Negative Outcome group was characterized by intraindividual elevations on the Conduct (36%) and Delinquency (55%) Scales which were elevated in only 20% of the Optimal Outcome group at admission.

## DISCUSSION

The dual criterion approach to treatment outcome evaluation provides simple, explicit and methodologically sound decision rules for categorizing clinical outcomes. The approach capitalizes on the strengths of both the statistical significance and clinical meaningfulness approaches considered singly. By considering statistical significance first, the model avoids interpreting changes that may reflect nothing more than chance variation or statistical artifact. The subsequent determination of the clinical meaningfulness of the change provides essential feedback about the impact of treatment on the client's functioning; an essential consideration in outcome research. The five operationally defined categories of clinical outcome also provide richer and more clinically useful information than the dichotomous outcome of significance testing.

Exploration of the differences in client variables among the various outcome groups can generate clinical hypotheses related to clinical course and may help identify positive prognostic indicators or risk factors. Finally, the approach lends itself well to continuous quality improvement efforts.

We hope that the treatment outcome evaluation methodology presented in the Devereux Scales of Mental Disorders and outlined in this article will provide professionals with a practical, technologically sound, and clinically useful tool to measure client outcomes in residential treatment centers and other mental health treatment settings.

## REFERENCES

American Psychiatric Association. (1994). *Diagnostic and statistical manual of mental disorders (4th ed.).* Washington, DC: Author.

Atkinson, L. (1991). Three standard errors of measurement and the Wechsler Memory Scale-Revised. *Psychological Assessment, 3,* 136-138.

Bednar, R.L., & Shapiro, J.B. (1970). Professional research commitment: A symptom or a syndrome? *Journal of Consulting and Clinical Psychology, 34,* 323-326.

Jacobsen, N.S., & Truax, P. (1991). Clinical significance: A statistical approach to defining meaningful change in psychotherapy research. *Journal of Consulting and Clinical Psychology, 59,* 12-19.

Linder, J.C. (1991). Outcomes measurement: Compliance tool or strategic initiative? *Health Care Management Review, 4,* 21-33.

Lord, F.M., & Novick, M.R. (1968). *Statistical theories of mental test scores.* Reading, MA: Addison-Wesley.

Mirin, S.M. & Namerow, M.J. (1991). Why study treatment outcome? *Hospital and Community Psychiatry, 10,* 1007-1013.

Naglieri, J.A., LeBuffe, P.A., & Pfeiffer, S.I. (1994). *The Devereux Scales of Mental Disorders.* San Antonio, TX: The Psychological Corporation.

O'Leary, D.S. (1993). The measurement mandate: Report card day is coming. *Journal for Quality Improvement, 19,* 487-491.

Pfeiffer, S.I. (1992). Clinicians and research: Constraints on scholarly activity. *Residential Treatment for Children & Youth, 9,* 41-48.

Pfeiffer, S.I., Burd, S., & Wright, A. (1992). Clinicians and research: Recurring obstacles and some possible solutions. *Journal of Clinical Psychology, 9,* 140-145.

Pratt, S.I., & Moreland, K.L. (1995). Introduction to treatment outcome: Historical Perspectives and Current Issues.

# Index

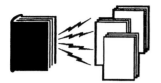

# Haworth
# DOCUMENT DELIVERY
# SERVICE

This valuable service provides a single-article order form for any article from a Haworth journal.

- *Time Saving:* No running around from library to library to find a specific article.
- *Cost Effective:* All costs are kept down to a minimum.
- *Fast Delivery:* Choose from several options, including same-day FAX.
- *No Copyright Hassles:* You will be supplied by the original publisher.
- *Easy Payment:* Choose from several easy payment methods.

> *Open Accounts Welcome for . . .*
> - Library Interlibrary Loan Departments
> - Library Network/Consortia Wishing to Provide Single-Article Services
> - Indexing/Abstracting Services with Single Article Provision Services
> - Document Provision Brokers and Freelance Information Service Providers

**MAIL or *FAX* THIS ENTIRE ORDER FORM TO:**

Haworth Document Delivery Service          **or FAX:** 1-800-895-0582
The Haworth Press, Inc.                    **or CALL:** 1-800-342-9678
10 Alice Street                                     9am-5pm EST
Binghamton, NY 13904-1580

PLEASE SEND ME PHOTOCOPIES OF THE FOLLOWING SINGLE ARTICLES:
1) Journal Title: _____
   Vol/Issue/Year: _____ Starting & Ending Pages: _____
   Article Title: _____

2) Journal Title: _____
   Vol/Issue/Year: _____ Starting & Ending Pages: _____
   Article Title: _____

3) Journal Title: _____
   Vol/Issue/Year: _____ Starting & Ending Pages: _____
   Article Title: _____

4) Journal Title: _____
   Vol/Issue/Year: _____ Starting & Ending Pages: _____
   Article Title: _____

**(See other side for Costs and Payment Information)**

*COSTS:* Please figure your cost to order quality copies of an article.

1. Set-up charge per article: $8.00
   ($8.00 × number of separate articles) _____

2. Photocopying charge for each article:
   1-10 pages: $1.00 _____

   11-19 pages: $3.00 _____

   20-29 pages: $5.00 _____

   30+ pages: $2.00/10 pages _____

3. Flexicover (optional): $2.00/article _____

4. Postage & Handling: US: $1.00 for the first article/
   $.50 each additional article _____

   Federal Express: $25.00 _____

   Outside US: $2.00 for first article/
   $.50 each additional article _____

5. Same-day FAX service: $.35 per page _____

### GRAND TOTAL: _____

---

*METHOD OF PAYMENT:* (please check one)
❏ Check enclosed     ❏ Please ship and bill. PO # _____
       (sorry we can ship and bill to bookstores only! All others must pre-pay)
❏ Charge to my credit card: ❏ Visa;  ❏ MasterCard;  ❏ Discover;
                  ❏ American Express;

Account Number: _____  Expiration date: _____

Signature: ✗ _____

Name: _____  Institution: _____

Address: _____

_____

City: _____  State: _____ Zip: _____

Phone Number: _____  FAX Number: _____

### MAIL or *FAX* THIS ENTIRE ORDER FORM TO:

| Haworth Document Delivery Service | **or FAX:** 1-800-895-0582 |
| The Haworth Press, Inc. | **or CALL:** 1-800-342-9678 |
| 10 Alice Street | 9am-5pm EST) |
| Binghamton, NY 13904-1580 | |

# DATE DUE